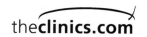

ENDOCRINOLOGY AND METABOLISM CLINICS
OF NORTH AMERICA

Impaired Glucose Tolerance and Cardiovascular Disease

GUEST EDITORS
Willa A. Hsueh, MD
Preethi Srikanthan, MD
Christopher J. Lyon, PhD

CONSULTING EDITOR
Derek LeRoith, MD, PhD

September 2006 • Volume 35 • Number 3

SAUNDERS

An Imprint of Elsevier, Inc.
PHILADELPHIA   LONDON   TORONTO   MONTREAL   SYDNEY   TOKYO

W.B. SAUNDERS COMPANY
A Division of Elsevier Inc.

1600 John F. Kennedy Boulevard • Suite 1800 • Philadelphia, Pennsylvania 19103-2899

http://www.theclinics.com

ENDOCRINOLOGY AND METABOLISM
CLINICS OF NORTH AMERICA
September 2006
Editor: Rachel Glover

Volume 35, Number 3
ISSN 0889-8529
ISBN 1-4160-3518-4

The ideas and opinions expressed in *Endocrinology and Metabolism Clinics of North America* do not necessarily reflect those of the Publisher. The Publisher does not assume any responsibility for any injury and/or damage to persons or property arising out of or related to any use of the material contained in this periodical. The reader is advised to check the appropriate medical literature and the product information currently provided by the manufacturer of each drug to be administered to verify the dosage, the method and duration of administration, or contraindications. It is the responsibility of the treating physician or other health care professional, relying on independent experience and knowledge of the patient, to determine drug dosages and the best treatment for the patient. Mention of any product in this issue should not be construed as endorsement by the contributors, editors, or the Publisher of the product or manufacturers' claims.

Endocrinology and Metabolism Clinics of North America (ISSN 0889-8529) is published quarterly by Elsevier Inc., 360 Park Avenue South, New York, NY 10010-1710. Months of publication are March, June, September, and December. Business and editorial offices: 1600 John F. Kennedy Boulevard, Suite 1800, Philadelphia, PA 19103-2899. Customer Service Office: 6277 Sea Harbor Drive, Orlando, FL 32887-4800. Periodicals postage paid at New York, NY and additional mailing offices. Subscription prices are USD 175 per year for US individuals, USD 295 per year for US institutions, USD 90 per year for US students and residents, USD 220 per year for Canadian individuals, USD 355 per year for Canadian institutions, USD 240 per year for international individuals, USD 355 per year for international institutions and USD 125 per year for Canadian and foreign students/residents. To receive student/resident rate, orders must be accompanied by name of affiliated institution, date of term, and the *signature* of program/residency coordinator on institution letterhead. Orders will be billed at individual rate until proof of status is received. Foreign air speed delivery is included in all *Clinics* subscription prices. All prices are subject to change without notice. POSTMASTER: Send address changes to *Endocrinology and Metabolism Clinics of North America*, Elsevier Periodicals Customer Service, 6277 Sea Harbor Drive, Orlando, FL 32887-4800. **Customer Service: (+1) 800-654-2452 (US). From outside of the US, call (+1) 407-345-4000; e-mail: hhspcs@harcourt.com.**

Reprints. For copies of 100 or more, of articles in this publication, please contact the Commercial Rights Department, Elsevier Inc., 360 Park Avenue South, New York, NY 10010-1710; phone: (+1) 212-633-3813; fax: (+1) 212-462-1935; e-mail: reprints@elsevier.com.

Endocrinology and Metabolism Clinics of North America is covered in *Index Medicus, EMBASE/Excerpta Medica, Current Contents/Clinical Medicine, Current Contents/Life Sciences, Science Citation Index, ISI/BIOMED, BIOSIS, and Chemical Abstracts.*

Printed in the United States of America.

CONSULTING EDITOR

DEREK LeROITH, MD, PhD, Chief, Division of Endocrinology, Metabolism, and Bone Diseases, Mount Sinai School of Medicine, New York, New York

GUEST EDITORS

WILLA A. HSUEH, MD, Professor of Medicine and Chief, Division of Endocrinology, Diabetes and Hypertension, David Geffen School of Medicine, University of California, Los Angeles, California

PREETHI SRIKANTHAN, MD, Assistant Clinical Professor, Department of Epidemiology and Preventative Medicine, University of California Los Angeles, Los Angeles, California

CHRISTOPHER J. LYON, PhD, Assistant Researcher, Division of Endocrinology, Diabetes and Hypertension, David Geffen School of Medicine, University of California Los Angeles, Los Angeles, California

CONTRIBUTORS

FLORIAN BLASCHKE, MD, Division of Endocrinology, Diabetes and Hypertension, David Geffen School of Medicine, University of California, Los Angeles, California

RAMANDEEP BRAR, MD, Clinical Cardiac Electrophysiology Fellow, UCLA Cardiac Arrhythmia Center, Division of Cardiology, Department of Medicine, David Geffen School of Medicine at UCLA, Los Angeles, California

EVREN CAGLAYAN, MD, Division of Endocrinology, Diabetes and Hypertension, David Geffen School of Medicine, University of California, Los Angeles, California

DAVID A. CESARIO, MD, PhD, Assistant Professor of Medicine, UCLA Cardiac Arrhythmia Center, Division of Cardiology, Department of Medicine, David Geffen School of Medicine at UCLA, Los Angeles, California

TINA J. CHAHIL, MD, Department of Medicine, College of Physicians and Surgeons of Columbia University, New York, New York

MARK E. COOPER, MBBS, PhD, Professor of Medicine; and Director, Vascular Division, Baker Heart Research Institute, Danielle Memorial Centre for Diabetes Complications, Wynn Domain, Melbourne, Victoria, Australia

JATIN K. DAVE, MD, MPH, Instructor in Medicine, Harvard Medical School, Division of Aging, Brigham and Women's Hospital, Boston, Massachusetts

SUSAN DAVIS, MD, Associate Clinical Professor, Department of Endocrinology, Diabetes and Metabolism, University of California Los Angeles, Los Angeles, California

GREGG C. FONAROW, MD, FACC, Eliot Corday Professor of Cardiovascular Medicine and Science Director, Ahmanson-UCLA Cardiomyopathy Center, UCLA Division of Cardiology, David Geffen School of Medicine at UCLA, Los Angeles, California

HENRY N. GINSBERG, MD, Department of Medicine, College of Physicians and Surgeons of Columbia University, New York, New York

MARTIN M. HARTGE, BPharm, Pharmacist, Center for Cardiovascular Research, Institute for Pharmacology, Charité Berlin, Berlin, Germany

KEVAN HEROLD, MD, Associate Professor of Medicine, Columbia University Medical Center, New York, New York

WILLA A. HSUEH, MD, Professor of Medicine and Chief, Division of Endocrinology, Diabetes and Hypertension, David Geffen School of Medicine, University of California, Los Angeles, California

KARIN JANDELEIT-DAHM, MD, PHD, Consultant Nephrologist; and Senior Research Fellow, Baker Heart Research Institute, Danielle Memorial Centre for Diabetes Complications, Wynn Domain, Melbourne, Victoria, Australia

VIKRAM V. KAMDAR, MD, Clinical Associate Professor of Medicine, David Geffen School of Medicine at UCLA, Santa Monica UCLA Medical Center, Santa Monica, California

ULRICH KINTSCHER, MD, Medical Doctor, Center for Cardiovascular Research, Institute for Pharmacology, Charité Berlin, Berlin, Germany

STANLEY KORENMAN, MD, Professor, Department of Endocrinology, Diabetes and Metabolism, University of California Los Angeles, Los Angeles, California

RAVICHANDRAN RAMSAMY, PhD, Assistant Professor of Surgery, Columbia University Medical Center, New York, New York

PETER D. REAVEN, MD, Director, Diabetes Program, Division of Endocrinology, Carl T. Hayden VA Medical Center, Phoenix, Arizona

ANN MARIE SCHMIDT, MD, Professor of Surgery, Columbia University Medical Center, New York, New York

ERIC A. SCHWARTZ, PhD, Research Health Scientist, Division of Research, Carl T. Hayden VA Medical Center, Phoenix, Arizona

KALYANAM SHIVKUMAR, MD, PhD, Director, UCLA Cardiac Arrhythmia Center and EP Program, Division of Cardiology, Department of Medicine, David Geffen School of Medicine at UCLA, Los Angeles, California

PREETHI SRIKANTHAN, MD, Assistant Clinical Professor, Department of Epidemiology and Preventative Medicine, University of California Los Angeles, Los Angeles, California

THOMAS UNGER, MD, Professor of Medicine, Center for Cardiovascular Research, Institute for Pharmacology, Charité Berlin, Berlin, Germany

SHI DU YAN, MD, Associate Professor of Surgery and Pathology, Columbia University Medical Center, New York, New York

SHI FANG YAN, MD, Assistant Professor of Surgery, Columbia University Medical Center, New York, New York

CONTENTS

Hypertension is often associated clinically with diabetes as part of
the insulin-resistance syndrome or as a manifestation of renal
disease. Elevated systemic blood pressure accelerates micro- and
macrovascular complications in diabetes. Vasoactive hormone pathways including the renin-angiotensin-aldosterone system (RAAS)
appear to play a pivotal role in the pathogenesis and progression
of diabetic complications and possibly of diabetes itself. Recent
studies have increased our understanding of the complexity of
the RAAS with identification of new components of this cascade
including angiotensin-converting enzyme 2 and a putative renin
receptor. Agents that interrupt the RAAS confer end-organ protection in diabetes via hemodynamic and non-hemodynamic mechanisms. Trials are investigating the possible role of RAAS blockade in
the prevention of type 2 diabetes.

Type 2 diabetes mellitus is associated with a markedly increased
risk of cardiovascular disease. A complex dyslipidemia, which is
an integral part of the underlying insulin resistance in this group,
is a key to this increased risk. Increased secretion of VLDL from
the liver is a central feature of dyslipidemia and is linked significantly to the low HDL and abnormal LDL that are also present.

A number of physiologic and pharmacologic approaches are available and should be used aggressively to treat diabetic dyslipidemia.

The presence of elevated blood glucose levels characterizes the diabetic state. Hyperglycemia may be caused by a number of underlying factors; however, the consequences of chronically elevated glucose are similar. Both the macrovasculature and microvasculature are exquisitely sensitive to the long-term effects of elevated blood glucose. Cardiovascular disease remains the leading cause of morbidity and mortality in diabetes, regardless of the underlying cause of hyperglycemia. Although other substrates, such as DNA, are susceptible to glycation, this article addresses the impact of nonenzymatic glycation on the proteome. The impact of Advanced Glycation End products (AGEs) on alteration of protein function and signal transduction mechanisms contributes to the pathogenesis of diabetes complications. This suggests that blocking the generation or molecular impact of AGEs may modulate the complications of diabetes.

Although the prevalence of cardiovascular complications is increased in insulin-resistant individuals, the underlying causes of this link have been elusive. Recent work suggests that several intracellular signal transduction pathways are inappropriately activated by hyperinsulinemia, hyperglycemia, increased free fatty acids, dyslipidemia, various inflammatory cytokines, and adipokines—factors that are increased in insulin resistance. Once activated, substantial cross talk occurs between these pathways, especially through reactive oxygen species-mediated mechanisms that induce a self-reinforcing cascade of vascular inflammation and cell dysfunction, greatly increasing the risk and severity of atherosclerosis in the insulin-resistant individual. We review several key cell-signaling pathways, describe how they are activated in the insulin-resistant state and the damage they induce, and discusses possible therapeutic approaches to limit vascular damage.

When normal endothelial function is shifted to a pathological degree, the foundation is laid for possibly following diseases. This endothelial dysfunction is characterized by a proinflammatory state, reduced vasodilation, and a prothrombotic state. In the continuation this dysfunction is strongly associated cardiovascular morbidity and mortality. Endothelial dysfunction is markedly enhanced in type 2 diabetes providing a major pathophysiological cause for the massively increased cardiovascular risk of diabetic patients. Subsequently future therapeutic approaches for the treatment of diabetic cardiovascular disease should target the dysfunctional endothelium first.

cardiomyopathy. This article initially gives some general background on diabetic cardiomyopathy and ion channels. Next the focus is on how diabetic cardiomyopathy alters calcium homeostasis in cardiac myocytes and highlights the specific alterations in ion channel function that are characteristic of this type of cardiomyopathy. Finally, the importance of the renin-angiotensin system in diabetic cardiomyopathy is reviewed.

All of the known risks for cardiovascular disease are increased in women with polycystic ovary syndrome, which features amenorrhea, hirsutism, and obesity. Epidemiologic studies in these patients and their families have revealed a familial predisposition not only to polycystic ovary syndrome, but also diabetes, hypertension, and cardiovascular disease. The heterogeneity of the phenotypes (clinically and biochemically) leads to difficulty in achieving a precise diagnosis, defining a single underlying pathogenesis, and selecting a homogeneous population for much needed prospective studies. The authors believe that while insulin resistance plays an important role in some cases of polycystic ovarian syndrome, it is the overall milieu created by the co-existence of several cardiovascular risk factors in polycystic ovarian syndrome patients which should be an important target for preventative strategies and therapy.

Ethnicity is a complex yet important construct and an independent risk factor for diabetic heart disease (DHD) with paramount clinical significance. Clinicians should try to better understand the role of ethnicity through more questions. The risk of DHD is modified by ethnicity, and its management may require a culturally sensitive individualized approach. Findings from Caucasian populations cannot be fully extrapolated to other ethnic groups, thereby emphasizing the importance of future research with ethnicity-specific data. Clinicians should be aware of an ethnicity-based threshold for obesity. Available limited data support the interaction between genetic predisposition, environmental risk, and lifestyle choices and disparities based on ethnicity as the likely cause for ethnic variations in DHD.

FORTHCOMING ISSUES

RECENT ISSUES

THE CLINICS ARE NOW AVAILABLE ONLINE!

Access your subscription at:
http://www.theclinics.com

ELSEVIER
SAUNDERS

Endocrinol Metab Clin N Am
35 (2006) xiii–xv

ENDOCRINOLOGY
AND METABOLISM
CLINICS
OF NORTH AMERICA

Foreword

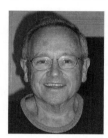

Derek LeRoith, MD, PhD
Consulting Editor

Understanding the relationship between impaired glucose tolerance and cardiovascular disease is clearly of paramount importance to internists, endocrinologists, and cardiologists for academic as well as practical reasons. Nobody is better qualified to deal with these issues than Willa Hsueh and her colleague Preethi Srikanthan, who have assembled a number of excellent reviews for this issue.

Eric Schwartz and Peter Reaven discuss the cellular mechanisms involved in the effects of insulin resistance on vascular cells. Insulin resistance is commonly associated with hyperglycemia and elevated free fatty acids, which can stimulate signaling pathways involved in the disease process affecting vascular smooth muscle cells (VSMCs), including nuclear factor kappa B (NF-κB), protein kinase C, and mitogen-activated protein kinase (MAPK). Reactive oxygen species (ROS) production may play a central role in the negative effects on VSMCs. These authors also address the effects of inflammation in different organs, such as fat, with release of adipocytokines that may initiate many of these deleterious effects.

The formation of advanced glycosylation end products (AGE), especially proteins, their interaction with the AGE receptor (RAGE) for these altered proteins, and their role in diabetic complications are discussed by Ann Marie Schmidt and colleagues. Although hyperglycemia is the primary cause of increased AGE products, the effects of AGE products on VSMCs include ROS production and upregulation of the expression of VCAM-1 and activation of NF-κB, all regulators of VSMC disordered function that potentially result in the vascular complications associated with hyperglycemia.

0889-8529/06/$ - see front matter © 2006 Elsevier Inc. All rights reserved.
doi:10.1016/j.ecl.2006.08.002   *endo.theclinics.com*

Diabetic dyslipidemia is clearly a cause of cardiovascular complications. Chahil and Ginsburg describe in detail normal lipid homeostasis as well as the abnormalities that occur in diabetes, focusing on type 2 diabetes but also indicating the abnormal changes seen in type 1 diabetes. As they point out, the major abnormality is overproduction of very low-density lipoprotein cholesterol, which accounts for the hypertriglyceridemia and low high-density lipoprotein levels that are commonly seen in patients with type 2 diabetes. They also address management, and stress that statins and fibrates are important therapeutic agents, but add that niacin is extremely useful, especially if the hyperglycemia is adequately controlled.

Unger and colleagues introduce their article with a discussion of the normal function of the endothelial cell, followed by an exploration of the abnormalities seen in diabetes as a result of metabolic disorders and inflammatory changes that are now commonly associated with obesity and diabetes. A central theme is the importance of nitric oxide, a molecule important in endothelial function and dysfunction. Endothelial dysfunction is characterized by reduced vasodilatation, a pro-inflammatory and a pro-thrombotic state. The authors also present evidence that thiazolidinediones maybe useful in correcting endothelial dysfunction and in reducing cardiovascular abnormalities in diabetics.

As described by Cooper and colleagues, the renin-aldosterone system (RAS) plays a central role in diabetes and its complications. Hypertension is extremely common in diabetic patients and has been attributed to the effects of insulin on renal salt handling, on the VSMCs via MAPK, and on the sympathetic nervous system. On the other hand, the RAS may play a role in increasing insulin resistance. Numerous studies have demonstrated that inhibition of the RAS using either angiotensin-converting enzyme (ACE) inhibition or angiotensin II receptor blockers is a powerful means of treating hypertension in diabetics, retarding diabetic nephropathy, and even preventing or delaying the development of type 2 diabetes in patients with impaired glucose tolerance. Whether these agents also retard retinopathy is as yet unclear, but ongoing clinical trials may yet prove this important function.

The relationship between diabetes and macrovascular complications including coronary artery disease is well recognized. Less well recognized is the entity of diabetic cardiomyopathy, an important cause of heart failure in these patients, discussed in the article by Gregg Fonarow and Preethi Srikanthan. The underlying pathophysiology is thought to include micrangiopathy, autonomic neuropathy, and metabolic factors described in the earlier articles. Most important, the authors point out, are the therapeutic options that include the use of beta blockers and ACE inhibitiors with concomitant glycemic control.

David Cesario, Ramandeep Brar, and Kalyanam Shivkumar describe the underlying mechanisms involved in diabetic cardiomyopathy, namely, the role of ion channels and altered calcium homeostasis. They hypothesize that in addition to the standard therapies, insulin-like growth factor-1 maybe a useful therapeutic agent, inasmuch as it has been shown experimentally to restore normal calcium homeostasis in diabetic cardiomyocytes, prevent the decline in sarco/endoplasmic reticulum CA^{2+} ATPase levels, promote cardiac growth, increase cardiac contractility, and increase cardiac output and ejection volume.

The influence of ethnicity on diabetic complications is extremely important, and Jatin Dave and Vikram Kamdar address the role of ethnicity in diabetic heart disease. Obesity, metabolic syndrome, impaired glucose tolerance, and diabetes are common in African Americans, Hispanic Americans, and Native Americans, and are becoming a problem in Asian Americans. Genetics is an obvious element in this high incidence of these various metabolic abnormalities, as well as environmental factors, and thus, studying the ethnic variations in predisposing factors to diabetic complications is an essential component for disease prevention and treatment.

Polycystic ovarian syndrome (PCOS) is a common cause of infertility but is also a classic example of hyperinsulinemia and insulin resistance. Therefore, Preethi Srikanthan, Stanley Korenman, and Susan Davis discuss the possibility that PCOS predisposes to cardiovascular complications. Although the evidence is gradually accumulating, it is important to consider this complication and treat the disorder appropriately both from a menstrual and infertility aspect and from the aspect of insulin resistance and its predictable outcomes. Metformin and thiazolidinediones have been shown in clinical trials to be effective in treating both aspects.

Willa Hsueh and colleagues summarize the effects of thiazolidinediones on the vasculature in diabetics. Experimental and clinical studies have demonstrated the value of these agents, not just as insulin sensitizers and in improving glucose homeostasis but also as protective to the vasculature at various stages of the disease process. The data suggest that some of the effects may be via insulin sensitivity and others may be directly on the inflammatory process that is commonly seen in obesity and type 2 diabetes. From many aspects, these agents have found an important role in managing diabetes and in preventing the deterioration of the cardiovascular complications.

This issue has focused on one major complication of diabetes, a common and devastating disease, and the issue editors and authors are to be commended for their focused articles that will ensure easy reading and a comprehensive reference for all practitioners.

Derek Leroith, MD, PhD
Division of Endocrinology and Diabetes
Department of Medicine
Mount Sinai School of Medicine
One Gustave L. Levy Place, Box 1055
Annenberg Building, Room 23-66B
New York, NY 10029-6574, USA

E-mail address: derek.leroith@mssm.edu

ELSEVIER
SAUNDERS

Endocrinol Metab Clin N Am
35 (2006) xvii–xix

ENDOCRINOLOGY
AND METABOLISM
CLINICS
OF NORTH AMERICA

Preface

Diabetes has a profoundly deleterious effect on the cardiovascular system. However, the pathophysiologic mechanisms, which commence even before the blood glucose threshold for diagnosis of diabetes is reached, are not well understood. Elucidation of these mechanisms is critically important to developing appropriate prevention and therapeutic strategies. The purpose of this edition of the *Endocrinology and Metabolism Clinics of North America* is to shed light on these multiple and complex mechanisms. Hypertension, dyslipidemia, hyperglycemia, and endothelial dysfunction are all key components of the metabolic syndrome. Hypertension exacerbates all macro- and microvascular complications of diabetes, and there is evidence of increased sensitivity to the renin-angiotensin-aldosterene system (RAAS) in diabetes, particularly in type 2, because adipose tissue is a source of the angiotension II precursor, angiotensinogen. In this issue, Jandeleit-Dahm and Cooper discuss evidence that RAAS inhibition attenuates diabetes complications and focus on new approaches to inhibiting this key system. Chahil and Ginsberg present a comprehensive analysis of lipoprotein metabolism in patients with type 1 and type 2 diabetes compared with normal subjects, and they suggest that overproduction of very low-density lipoprotein is a central feature leading to lower high-density lipoprotein cholesterol levels and more small, compacted low-density lipoprotein cholesterol, which is highly atherogenic because of its propensity toward oxidation. Yan and colleagues discuss evidence that glucose promotes cardiovascular complications by the formation of advanced glycosylation end products (AGEs) that promote inflammation, oxidation, and alter protein function and cell signaling pathways to damage tissues. They highlight the protective effects of blocking the AGE receptor (RAGE) using soluble RAGE. Schwartz and Reaven expand on the role of alterations in key cell signaling pathways and the critical

doi:10.1016/j.ecl.2006.08.001   *endo.theclinics.com*

intersection of these alterations with oxidative stress, leading to a complex network of vascular injury. They discuss novel approaches to correct these alterations. The endothelium is a major protector of the vasculature. Hartge and colleagues discuss detailed mechanisms by which the endothelial barrier is destroyed in insulin resistance and diabetes and how activation of the nuclear receptor peroxisome proliferator-activated receptor gamma (PPARγ) may protect the endothelium. Finally, Blaschke and colleagues amplify the discussion of the potential vasoprotective effects of PPARγ ligands, focusing on mechanisms of protection as well as side effects of the ligands.

The heart is also a key target of damage in diabetes. Fonarow and Srikanthan define diabetic cardiomyopathy and discuss in detail the mechanisms of cardiac damage in diabetes. Many of the mechanisms that damage the heart are the same as those that damage the vasculature, but also include widespread microangiopathy and autonomic neuropathy. These authors highlight the clinical presentation of diabetic cardiomyopathy and discuss recommended and potential novel therapies. Cesario and colleagues focus on a topic that is important, however infrequently discussed—channel alterations in diabetic cardiomyopathy. They discuss altered calcium homeostasis and how current and newly proposed therapies may improve these alterations.

This issue concludes with a focus on populations vulnerable to cardiovascular disease. Dave and Kamdar comprehensively review data on the influence of ethnicity on the risk of developing diabetes and diabetes associated cardiovascular disease. Of note, non-Hispanic Whites generally have lower rates of obesity and metabolic syndrome, but higher rates of diabetic heart disease. An increasingly important, but complex issue in women is polycytic ovarian syndrome (PCOS). Srikanthan and colleagues discuss pathophysiology of the hormone abnormalities and their relationship to hyperinsulinemia and insulin resistance. Finally, they outline potential mechanisms leading to increased cardiovascular disease risk and approaches to prevention and treatment of the same.

Despite several decades of promising research, cardiovascular disease remains the number one cause of mortality in men and women in the United States. Thankfully, there is widespread public recognition of the importance of factors involved in cardiovascular disease prevention (as first illustrated by the Framingham study). However, this issue of *Endocrinology and Metabolism Clinics of North America* highlights the contribution of several different events (such as hypertension, dyslipidemia, formation of advanced glycosylation end products and endothelial dysfunction) accompanying and leading to glucose intolerance, and of related conditions (such as diabetic cardiomyopathy and PCOS) to cardiovascular risk. Additionally, in a multi-ethnic society such the United States today, it is of vital importance to recognize the effect of race on cardiovascular disease risk. Hence, as we face an epidemic of obesity and type 2 diabetes, it is imperative that we reflect on how knowledge of these factors should alter and improve our approach to cardiovascular disease prevention and therapy.

Willa A. Hsueh, MD
Division of Endocrinology, Diabetes, and Hypertension
University of California Los Angeles
900 Veteran Avenue, Suite 24-130
Los Angeles, CA 90095, USA

E-mail address: whsueh@mednet.ucla.edu

Preethi Srikanthan, MD
Department of Epidemiology and Preventative Medicine
University of California Los Angeles
330 S. Garfield Avenue, Suite 308
Alhambra, CA 91801, USA

E-mail address: psrikanthan@mednet.ucla.edu

Christopher J. Lyon, PhD
Division of Endocrinology, Diabetes and Hypertension
University of California Los Angeles
900 Veteran Avenue, Suite 24-130
Los Angeles, CA 90095, USA

E-mail address: clyon@mednet.ucla.edu

ELSEVIER
SAUNDERS

Endocrinol Metab Clin N Am
35 (2006) 469–490

ENDOCRINOLOGY
AND METABOLISM
CLINICS
OF NORTH AMERICA

Hypertension and Diabetes: Role of the Renin-Angiotensin System

Karin Jandeleit-Dahm, MD, PhD,
Mark E. Cooper, MBBS, PhD*

*Baker Heart Research Institute, Danielle Memorial Centre for Diabetes Complications,
Wynn Domain, 75 Commercial Road, Melbourne 3004, Victoria, Australia*

Diabetes and hypertension are comorbid diseases that independently predispose to renal and cardiovascular complications. Both diseases exacerbate each other in terms of subsequent renal and cardiovascular complications [1]. Although effective antihypertensive agents are available, achieving adequate blood pressure control remains difficult in hypertensive patients, particularly in the context of concomitant diabetes. Although β-blockers and diuretics have been the most commonly used combination in the treatment of hypertension, there has recently been increasing reticence to use these agents, particularly in combination, because of metabolic side effects and probably reduced end-organ protection when compared with newer antihypertensive agents. It remains unresolved as to whether blood pressure reduction per se is the most important target of antihypertensive treatment or if there are specific benefits associated with certain antihypertensive regimens, in particular inhibitors of the renin-angiotensin—aldosterone system (RAAS). Already in the diabetic setting, agents that interrupt the renin-angiotensin system and increasingly also the aldosterone pathway appear to be particularly useful in diabetic renal and cardiovascular disease [2,3]. Retinopathy also appears to be an appropriate target for agents that modulate the renin-angiotensin system but this role remains unproven [4].

Because most patients with diabetes and hypertension will require more than 2 or 3 antihypertensive drugs to achieve target blood pressures as recommended in the latest US, European, and World Health Organization

K.J.D. is a postdoctoral clinical fellow supported by the National Heart Foundation of Australia.
* Corresponding author.
E-mail address: mark.cooper@baker.edu.au (M.E. Cooper).

(WHO) guidelines the most beneficial combination of antihypertensive drugs still needs to be established. Here we will review potential new drug targets as a result of recent basic science discoveries related to the RAAS as well as critically analyzing evidence from recently published trials with a particular focus on combination treatment regimens.

Diabetes and hypertension: cause and consequence

Type 1 diabetes

In type 1 diabetes the onset of hypertension appears to occur primarily as a consequence rather than as a primary cause of renal disease [5]. With the onset of hypertension in type 1 diabetes, usually associated with microalbuminuria, there appears to be an acceleration in the development of microvascular complications including nephropathy and retinopathy. The link between hypertension and atherosclerosis in type 1 diabetes has not been as extensively characterized as in type 2 diabetes, but it is likely that the elevation in systemic blood pressure in this form of diabetes is also associated with increased macrovascular disease. The link between glycemic control and the development of hypertension has been demonstrated in the follow-up of the landmark Diabetes Control and Complications Trial (DCCT), the Epidemiology of Diabetes Interventions and Complications (EDIC) study [6]. It was specifically demonstrated that hypertension developed in 40% of the patients in the conventionally treated group compared with 30% in the group treated with an intensified insulin regimen at year 8 of the EDIC follow-up. These beneficial effects of intensified glycemic control were seen in the context of reduced renal disease consistent with the view that hypertension in type 1 diabetes is primarily a manifestation of diabetic nephropathy in these subjects. Furthermore, it has recently been shown that blood pressure improves in type 1 diabetic subjects after combined kidney/pancreas transplantation, a phenomenon that does not occur with kidney transplantation alone [7]. Therefore, it appears likely that hyperglycemia or insulin play a role in influencing blood pressure in type 1 diabetes [7].

Type 2 diabetes

It has been clearly shown epidemiologically that hypertension and type 2 diabetes appear to cluster clinically as part of a syndrome involving not only these two conditions but also insulin resistance, dyslipidemia, central obesity, hyperuricemia, and accelerated atherosclerosis [8–10]. The underlying explanation for this cluster of clinical features remains unexplained but insulin resistance has been postulated by many investigators to play a pivotal role [9]. Therefore, this syndrome has been described using a range of terms including insulin-resistance syndrome [8], the metabolic syndrome [11], or "syndrome X" [12].

Insulin resistance and hypertension

Insulin resistance is often present in individuals with so called " prediabetes" who have impaired fasting glucose levels as well as glucose intolerance, as documented by postprandial hyperglycaemia in response to an oral glucose challenge. This abnormality in glucose homeostasis represents a risk factor for cardiovascular disease, even in the absence of significant hyperglycemia [11]. As insulin resistance may lead to hyperglycemia and dyslipidemia, links between insulin resistance and vascular dysfunction are not totally unexpected. In addition, insulin resistance may directly induce hypertension. Indeed, it was reported almost 20 years ago that patients with essential hypertension have higher insulin levels than normotensive subjects with a direct correlation between insulin levels and blood pressure [13]. However, it remains unclear if hypertension per se can cause insulin resistance.

There are several explanations for the link between insulin resistance and hypertension. First, it has been suggested that angiotensin II (AII) is involved in the development of insulin resistance in particular in the context of hypertension with an increasing body of data reporting direct effects of AII on insulin signaling pathways [14].

Second, it has been suggested that insulin may alter renal handling of sodium, in particular via effects on tubular sodium handling and salt sensitivity [15]. Insulin signaling leading to its well-characterized metabolic actions is mediated via PI-3 kinase, whereas the mitogenic effects of insulin are via the extracellular signal-regulated kinase (ERK)-mitogen activated protein kinase (MAP) pathway. In insulin-resistance syndromes, a dissociation between the two major signaling pathways of insulin has been described [16]. While there is resistance to the metabolic actions of insulin, the signaling cascade via ERK on cellular proliferation and fibrosis is still intact and indeed may be enhanced in this hyperinsulinemic state. Insulin itself is a potent vasoactive substance mediating vasodilation via NO availability [17] and increasing vasoconstrictor activities including the sympathetic nervous system, angiotensin II, and endothelin-1 [18,19]. As the vasodilatory effects of insulin are mediated via the PI-3 kinase pathway, resistance to this signaling pathway will lead to an imbalance between vasodilatory and vasoconstrictory actions of insulin shifting toward increased vascular tone and contributing to endothelial dysfunction. Indeed, acute hyperinsulinemia has been reported to lead to an increase in blood pressure in type 2 diabetic patients [20], whereas there was no such effect of insulin in healthy subjects [21].

The renin-angiotensin-aldosterone system and diabetic nephropathy

Diabetes is the most common cause of end-stage renal disease in the Western world [22]. The RAAS and in particular its effector molecule, angiotensin II (AII), has a range of hemodynamic and nonhemodynamic effects that contribute not only to the development of hypertension but also to renal disease.

The status of the RAAS in the diabetic kidney remains controversial with evidence of reduced, unchanged, or increased levels or activity of various components of this pathway, including enzymes and receptors [23,24]. Furthermore, there may be a redistribution of components of the renin-angiotensin system (RAS) within the diabetic kidney. For example, ACE may be redistributed in diabetes to glomeruli [24], whereas renin and AII may be expressed de novo in proximal tubules in the diabetic kidney [25,26] with subsequent activation of prosclerotic cytokines such as transforming growth factor- β1 (TGF-β1) thereby inducing tubulointerstitial fibrosis.

Experimental studies in both normo- and hypertensive models of diabetic nephropathy have clearly demonstrated renoprotective effects of agents that interrupt the RAS including angiotensin-converting enzyme (ACE) inhibitors and angiotensin II type 1 (AT1) receptor blockers (ARBs) [27]. With the increasing evidence of nonhemodynamic effects of AII, a range of other effects relevant to preservation of renal function and structure have been described including effects on prosclerotic cytokines, extracellular matrix proteins, and various chemokines linked to macrophage infiltration and proliferation [28]. The reduction of the slit pore protein nephrin in diabetic nephropathy has been linked to the development of proteinuria and appears to be partly AII dependent. Indeed, treatment with ARBs in diabetic rats restored renal nephrin depletion in experimental diabetes [29].

Since AII stimulates aldosterone, a proven mediator of inflammation and fibrosis, this provides another mechanism whereby blockade of the RAAS could lead to reduced glomerulosclerosis and tubulointerstitial fibrosis [30]. Indeed, aldosterone appears, based predominantly on preclinical data, to be a powerful inducer of renal inflammation and injury. Furthermore, blockade of the actions of aldosterone using agents such as spironolactone attenuates various forms of progressive renal disease although diabetic nephropathy has not been as extensively investigated [30] . The advent of the selective mineralocorticoid receptor antagonist eplerenone as well as new studies with spironolactone have stimulated investigation of the role of aldosterone in diabetic nephropathy (see aldosterone antagonists).

Prorenin activation

In diabetes, despite evidence of local activation of the RAS, plasma renin levels are low whereas plasma prorenin is elevated, a phenomenon that has been called the "diabetic paradox" [31]. Increased serum prorenin levels have been reported to predict microvascular complications and indeed often precede the onset of microalbuminuria [32]. When diabetes is induced in transgenic rats specifically overexpressing renin, the Ren2 rat, the severe structural changes in the kidney have marked resemblance to human diabetic nephropathy including the development of nodular sclerotic lesions, reminiscent of the Kimmelstiel-Wilson nodules seen in advanced diabetic nephropathy [33]. Recently, consistent with a role for renin in promoting diabetic nephropathy, it has been shown that inhibiting prorenin activation prevented streptozotocin-diabetes–induced glomerulosclerosis both acutely and in a chronic infusion model. Inhibition of prorenin activation was achieved by administering a "handle region protein" (HRP) working as a decoy that effectively competes for prorenin binding to its receptor [34]. Although the relevance in human diabetic nephropathy remains to be established, it may represent a novel target for the treatment and prevention of diabetic nephropathy, particularly in the context of concomitant hypertension. This area of research has been further stimulated by the discovery of various putative renin receptors or renin-binding proteins. These receptors bind both renin and prorenin and also lead to prorenin activation, either proteolytically or nonproteolytically. These findings may help to explain the predictive value of increased prorenin levels in diabetic subjects for the onset of microalbuminuria. Of particular interest is the recent identification of a putative renin receptor, which not only facilitates angiotensin generation but also leads to the activation of the mitogen-activated protein kinase (MAPK) pathway [35]. This indicates for the first time a direct, AII independent action of renin. The role of these putative renin receptors in diabetes remains to be ascertained. It will be of interest to investigate the role of the new renin inhibitors in diabetes and hypertension and to compare their effects with conventional blockade of the RAS. Furthermore, it is anticipated that novel drug treatments will be derived from this research such as specific renin receptor blockers that will specifically inhibit renin-mediated AII formation or signaling pathways in tissues [31].

Angiotensin-converting enzyme and angiotensin-converting enzyme 2

ACE plays a critical role in formation of AII but is not considered a major rate-limiting step in the RAAS. ACE inhibitors are widely prescribed in diabetic patients but abnormalities in ACE per se are not considered to play a central role in diabetic nephropathy and other complications. However, certain ACE gene polymorphisms have been linked not only to progression of diabetic nephropathy but also to response to ACE inhibitors [36]. Nevertheless, these findings have not been universal. It is interesting that recent experimental studies by our own group have emphasized the possibility of increased intravascular expression and activity of ACE in diabetes-associated atherosclerosis. The relevance of these findings to the clinical context is as yet unknown.

The classical view of the renin-angiotensin-aldosterone cascade has been increasingly challenged with the discovery of new components such as the enzyme ACE2 (Fig. 1). This enzyme with homology to ACE, is expressed in the heart and kidney consistent with a role for this enzyme in renal and

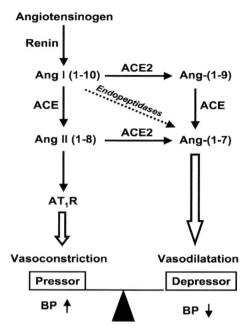

Fig. 1. New concept of the renin angiotensin system: balance between vasoconstriction and vasodilatation. Ang, angiotensin; ACE, angiotensin-converting enzyme; BP, blood pressure; AT_1R, angiotensin type 1 receptor.

cardiovascular physiology [37]. ACE2 only has a single catalytic site and catalyzes the cleavage of Angiotensin I (A1-10) into Angiotensin 1-9, which can further be cleaved by ACE to Angiotensin 1-7. Furthermore, AII can be converted directly by ACE2 to A1-7. A1-7 has been shown to exert vasodilatory properties and to antagonize the vasoconstriction mediated by AII, thereby contributing to the fine balance of vasodilators and vasoconstrictors generated by the various components of the renin-angiotensin system. Interestingly, ACE2 knockout mice demonstrate cardiac dysfunction thus illustrating the potential role of ACE2 in cardiac disease [38]. The additional deletion of ACE in the ACE2 KO mouse reversed the cardiac abnormalities observed in the single mutant ACE2 knockout mouse. In a study by our group investigating the status of ACE and ACE2 in diabetic nephropathy, reduced tubular ACE2 protein expression in diabetes, which was normalized by ACE inhibitor treatment, was observed [39]. A reduction in renal ACE2 has been reported in two animal models of hypertension including the spontaneously hypertensive rat (SHR) [38]. The identification of ACE2 in the kidney [40] and modulation of this enzyme by diabetes provide further complexity to the nature and role of the various components of the renal and cardiovascular RAS. As ACE2 appears to play a significant role in the balance between vasodilators and vasoconstrictors in the kidney as well as in the cardiovascular system, this enzyme may become a target for the development of specific therapies that could be relevant to progressive renal disorders such as diabetic nephropathy and cardiovascular disease.

Clinical studies in diabetic nephropathy

Numerous studies identifying renoprotection in type 1 and 2 diabetes at various stages of nephropathy have been described over the past 20 years with landmark studies such as the Collaborative Study Group Trial using captopril [41] and the more recent studies with AT1 receptor antagonists such as the Reduction of Endpoints in NIDDM with the Angiotensin II Antagonist Losartan (RENAAL) [42], Irbesartan Type 2 Diabetic Nephropathy Trial (IDNT) [43], and IRbesartan MicroAlbuminuria type 2 diabetes mellitus in hypertensive patients (IRMA-2) trials [44]. Subsequent meta-analyses such as one analyzing 12 placebo-controlled trials in 698 normotensive type 1 diabetic patients with microalbuminuria treated with ACE inhibitors [45] have further strengthened the evidence for a renoprotective role for agents that interrupt the RAS, even in the absence of hypertension.

A major issue remains whether there is a difference between ACE inhibition and AII receptor antagonism in terms of renal protection. Consistent with experimental evidence that AT1 receptor blockers provide equivalent renoprotection to ACE inhibitors in diabetes [46], a cross-over study of relatively short duration showed similar reductions in albuminuria with losartan and enalapril in type 1 diabetic subjects with macroproteinuria [47]. The more recently reported DETAIL study (Diabetics exposed to Telmisartan and Enalapril), a multicenter randomized, double-blind parallel-group trial, compared the AII antagonist, telmisartan, with the ACE inhibitor, enalapril, in 272 type 2 diabetic patients [48,49]. This study showed that the ARB telmisartan conferred similar renoprotection to the ACE inhibitor with a similar decline in glomerular filtration rate over 5 years in both groups. Ongoing studies comparing ARBs and ACE inhibitor treatments on renal and cardiovascular endpoints such as the Ongoing Telmisartan Alone and in Combination with Ramipril Global Endpoint Trial (ONTARGET) [50] and earlier commencement of ARBs before evidence of early or advanced renal disease such as the ROADMAP trial using olmesartan [51] should further assist in determining the appropriate role, dose and timing of ACE inhibitor or ARB in patients with or at risk of diabetic nephropathy (http://www.clinicaltrials.gov/ct/show/NCT00185159).

Aldosterone antagonists

Plasma aldosterone levels may not be abnormal in diabetic nephropathy but aldosterone blockade could potentially be renoprotective including in the context of diabetes. It has been suggested that reinfusion of aldosterone despite continued blockade of the renin-angiotensin system may promote renal fibrosis in hypertension [52].

The role of aldosterone antagonists including spironolactone and the more selective mineralocorticoid receptor antagonist eplerenone have been extensively examined over the past 5 years, albeit most of the studies have been of relatively short duration [2].

In type 2 diabetic patients with nephropathy, the aldosterone antagonist spironolactone added onto the maximal recommended dose of ACE inhibitor/ARB further reduced albuminuria. These effects were seen in the context of superior blood pressure reduction as assessed by 24-hour ambulatory blood pressure monitoring. However, the renal effects observed did not correlate with the effects on blood pressure [53]. In more recent short-term studies, the addition of spironolactone to existing antihypertensive medication including maximally recommended doses of ACE inhibitors/ARBs in type 1 [54] and type 2 diabetic patients [55] with diabetic nephropathy confirmed superior effects on albuminuria with a further reduction of 30% and a further decrease in blood pressure. Another study in type 2 diabetic patients with a follow-up of 1 year demonstrated a 44% further reduction in albuminuria in the group with added on spironolactone treatment. However, in that study this effect was at the expense of a faster rate of deterioration of renal function, although long-term detrimental effects on renal function appear to be unlikely [56].

The more selective mineralocorticoid receptor antagonist eplerenone, without anti-androgenic side effects such as gynecomastia was studied in type 2 diabetic patients with nephropathy in comparison to enalapril and as a combination regimen [57]. After 24 weeks, eplerenone monotherapy exceeded the ACE inhibitor monotherapy effect on proteinuria (62% versus 45% reduction in proteinuria). The combination treatment was associated with a 74% reduction in proteinuria, suggesting an additive or synergistic effect on proteinuria with both drugs. This antiproteinuric effect was associated with similar reductions in blood pressures suggesting an added possible blood pressure independent effect of mineralocorticoid receptor antagonism in this population.

Combination therapy

Most monotherapies do not appear to be able to lead to blood pressure levels as recommended in international guidelines (Seventh Report of the Joint National Committee on Prevention, Detection, Evaluation, and Treatment of High Blood Pressure and evidence from new hypertension trials, JNC-VII) [58], thus most diabetic patients will require combination regimens. It remains controversial as to which combination confers the optimal renoprotection and blood pressure control in patients with diabetic nephropathy.

The combination most often used is the addition of a diuretic to an ACE inhibitor or an ARB. The rationale behind this combination is, first, that the ACE inhibitor will counteract the activation of the RAS triggered by the diuretic and that, second, interruption of the RAS is more effective in lowering blood pressure in salt-depleted states. The PREMIER study (Preterax in Albuminuria Regression study) [59] compared the effect of low-dose perindopril/indapamide versus enalapril on albumin excretion in hypertensive, albuminuric type 2 diabetic patients. The combination resulted in greater antihypertensive and antiproteinuric effects. Furthermore a superior cardiovascular protection was observed in the combination group. However, this finding on cardiovascular outcomes was not a primary endpoint of the study and needs to be confirmed in larger prospective studies. The results of the ADVANCE study (Action in Diabetes and Vascular Disease: Preterax and Diamicron MR Controlled Evaluation) are now awaited comparing the effect of perindopril/indapamide or placebo on micro- and macrovascular outcomes in high-risk type 2 diabetic patients [60].

There is a small body of evidence to suggest that the combination of an ACE inhibitor or an ARB with a nondihydropyridine calcium channel blocker (ND-CCB) has superior effects on blood pressure control and proteinuria than monotherapies or combinations using dihydropyridine calcium channel blockers (D-CCB) [61]. The INVEST study (International Verapamil SR/Trandolapril study) [62] demonstrated that the combination of ND-CCB with an ACE inhibitor was as effective as β-blocker–based therapy in hypertensive diabetic subjects with coronary artery disease. More recently the Bergamo Nephrologic Diabetes Complications Trial (BENEDICT) compared the ACE inhibitor trandolapril and the nondihydropyridine CCB verapamil alone and in combination on the prevention of microalbuminuria in a cohort of 1204 patients with type 2 diabetes, hypertension but without albuminuria. The primary endpoint (development of albuminuria) was achieved in 5.7% in the combination group, 6% in the trandolapril group, compared with 11.9% in the verapamil group and 10% in the placebo group. These results suggest that ACE inhibitor alone or in combination with a nondihydropyridine CCB decreased the incidence of microalbuminuria in type 2 diabetic patients with hypertension [63].

The combination of an ACE inhibitor and an ARB promises a more complete blockade of the RAS potentially increasing the antihypertensive and renoprotective effects of both drugs. The Candesartan And Lisinopril Microalbuminuria (CALM) study demonstrated that the combination of an ACE inhibitor, lisinopril, and an AT1 receptor blocker, candesartan, was associated with improved blood pressure control and a trend toward reduced urinary albumin excretion when compared with either agent as monotherapy in a cohort of microalbuminuric hypertensive type 2 diabetic subjects [64]. A number of smaller studies, usually of short duration, have since demonstrated superior effects of the combination of two agents that interrupt the RAS compared with one agent alone on blood pressure and proteinuria in type 1 and 2 diabetic patients [65–67]. Furthermore, in three short-term cross-over studies in type 1 and 2 diabetic patients, dual blockade of the RAS by adding maximal recommended/effective doses of ARB or placebo to a maximal recommended dose of an ACE inhibitor has proven to be superior to maximal recommended doses of ACE inhibition alone on albuminuria and blood pressure [68–70]. The results of the CALM II study however are less convincing. In that study the antihypertensive and antiproteinuric effect of dual RAS blockade (candesartan cilexetil 16 mg and lisinopril 20 mg) with a higher ACE inhibitor dosage titration regimen (lisinopril 40 mg) in type 1 and 2 hypertensive diabetic patients over 12 months was examined [71]. The two treatments had similar effects on blood pressure and albumin/creatinine ratios. However, there were discrepancies in add-on thiazide treatment (higher in the dual blockade group) patients requiring additional antihypertensive therapy and withdrawals owing to persistently elevated blood pressures.

In all of these combination ACE inhibition/ARB studies it has remained difficult to determine if justifying higher doses of these agents, often not currently recommended, may lead to as good blood pressure control and renoprotection as the combinations. Indeed, a recent study by Parving's group using very high doses of irbesartan, up to 900 mg (3 times the recommended dose) showed the highest reduction in albuminuria in the ultrahigh-dose group compared with the lower dose groups (300 and 600 mg). This renoprotective effect in the ultrahigh-dose group (900 mg) was observed with no additional reduction in blood pressure suggesting a dose-dependent and blood pressure–independent effect in early diabetic nephropathy [72].

The Ongoing Telmisartan Alone and in Combination with Ramipril Global Endpoint Trial/ Telmisartan Randomized Assessment Study in ACE Intolerant Subjects with Cardiovascular Disease (ONTARGET/ TRANSCEND) trial [50] is comparing the ARB telmisartan with the ACE inhibitor ramipril as monotherapies and as a combination in high-risk patients with cardiovascular disease or diabetes with end-organ damage, similar to the study population in the Heart Outcomes Prevention Evaluation (HOPE) study [73]. The primary outcome is the composite of cardiovascular death, myocardial infarction, stroke, or hospitalization for heart failure. The results of such studies will help to identify the role of ACE inhibitors, ARBs, and their combination in prevention of cardiovascular endpoints in high-risk patients in the presence or absence of diabetes.

It remains to be fully delineated if the potential disadvantage of the dual blockade of the RAS, such as an increased risk of hyperkalemia and acute renal impairment, particularly in patients with renal artery stenosis, on cyclooxygenase-inhibitors, in salt- and fluid-depleted subjects or in patients with anemia may outweigh some of the renal and potential cardiovascular benefits seen with these regimens [74].

Heart failure and cardiovascular disease

The increased vascular disease in diabetes is clearly multifactorial with comorbid conditions such as hypertension possibly playing a greater role than metabolic factors in the predisposition and increased rate of progression of atherosclerosis in diabetes. In a recent population-based study, which involved transesophageal echocardiography to assess aortic atherosclerosis, diabetes was associated with an approximately 3-fold increase in atherosclerosis [75]. Interestingly, systolic blood pressure, pulse pressure, and age also correlated with atherosclerosis. It is likely that the increase in atherosclerosis in diabetic subjects may partly relate to these individuals often being older and having higher systolic and pulse pressures.

Diabetes is associated with left ventricular hypertrophy (LVH) [76]. This partly relates to the increased prevalence of hypertension [77] but also appears to be a diabetes-specific phenomenon that has been described by some investigators in association with functional abnormalities of the heart as "diabetic cardiomyopathy" [9]. In these individuals, the coronary arteries often do not have evidence of significant atherosclerosis. In these diabetic patients, as part of this cardiomyopathy, there is impaired diastolic function [78]. Hypertension exacerbates these cardiac abnormalities with evidence from the Strong Heart Study that the combination of diabetes and hypertension results in the greatest degree of LVH, myocardial dysfunction, and arterial stiffness [79]. Left ventricular systolic function was also particularly reduced in diabetes. A recent analysis from the large RENAAL study has further explored this issue. LVH was shown in that study to be significantly associated with the primary endpoint, which was a composite of the doubling of serum creatinine (DSCR) and progression to end-stage renal disease (ESRD) or death (hazard ratio = 1.44, P = .011) as well as the composite renal endpoint DSCR/ESRD (hazard ratio = 1.42, P = .031) and cardiovascular events (hazard ratio = 1.68, P = .001). Treatment with losartan reduced LVH by 6%, as diagnosed using electrocardiogram criteria. Furthermore, losartan treatment in these patients with type 2 diabetes, nephropathy, and LVH, reduced the cardiovascular and renal risk to levels similar to those observed in patients without LVH [80] (Fig. 2).

In the recently published Anglo-Scandinavian Cardiac Outcomes Trial (ASCOT) [81], which had the same endpoint as the very large Antihypertensive and Lipid-Lowering Treatment to Prevent Heart Attack (ALLHAT) trial [82,83] the hypothesis that newer drug combinations would confer superior reductions in blood pressure and superior cardiovascular protection compared with older drug combinations was examined. The rationale for this study was based on the shortfalls in prevention of cardiovascular disease in previous hypertensive trials that has been attributed to disadvantages of the diuretic-β-blocker combination. The ASCOT trial was a prospective, randomized trial including 19257 patients with hypertension aged 40 to 79 years with at least three other cardiovascular risk factors. Patients were

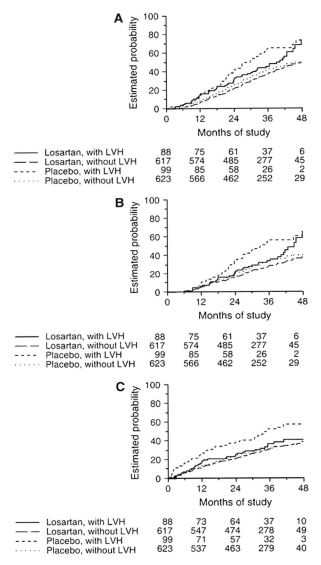

Fig. 2. Kaplan Meier estimates of the influence of left ventricular hypertrophy (LVH) and losartan-based therapy on (*A*) the primary composite endpoint of doubling of serum creatinine (DSCR), end-stage renal disease (ESRD) or death; (*B*) the renal composite endpoint of DSCR/ESRD; and (*C*) the cardiovascular morbidity and mortality composite endpoint. (*From* Boner G, Cooper ME, McCarroll K, et al. Adverse effects of left ventricular hypertrophy in the reduction of endpoints in NIDDM with the angiotensin II antagonist losartan (RENAAL) study. Diabetologia 2005;48:1984; with permission.).

assigned to either amlodipine 5 to 10 mg adding perindopril 4 to 8 mg or atenolol adding bendroflumethazole 1.25 to 2.5 mg. The primary endpoint was fatal myocardial infarction (MI) (including silent MI) and fatal coronary heart disease. The study was terminated prematurely after 5.5 years of follow-up as the amlodipine-perindopril group had less primary endpoint events. Major cardiovascular events were reduced by 16%, stroke by 23%, and cardiovascular as well as total mortality by 24% and 11% respectively [81].

It remains controversial as to whether the results of the ASCOT trial were a result of the better reduction in systolic blood pressure in the amlodipine/ perindopril group or of specific effects of the combinations on vascular or metabolic parameters [84]. Although some investigators have suggested that the better blood pressure reduction of 2.4 mm Hg in the CCB/ACE inhibitor group explained the beneficial cardiovascular outcomes, others have claimed that the reduction in cardiovascular outcomes exceeded that predicted from superior blood pressure reduction alone. This study included 27% diabetic patients in each treatment group but a specific subanalysis of the diabetic cohort has as yet not been published.

The underlying mechanisms for impaired cardiac function in the presence of hyperglycemia and specifically in the context of diabetes are now actively being investigated. This includes evidence of a role for the local RAAS in the heart, which appears to be activated in experimental diabetes [9]. In addition, changes in cellular hypertrophy, proliferation, and cell death including increased apoptosis in both experimental and human diabetic hearts [85], as well as changes in various trophic factors such as insulin-like growth factor-1 (IGF-1) and altered function of cationic channels and pumps may also be implicated in this "cardiomyopathy" of diabetes [9]. These recent experimental findings linking hyperglycemia and the RAAS to various pathways linked to cardiac remodeling provide the rationale for further clinical studies directly addressing the effects of intensified glycemic control and blockade of the RAAS on diabetes-associated LVH and diastolic dysfunction. In this context the results of the ONTARGET trial (see combination therapy) will help to identify the role of ACE inhibitors, ARBs, and their combination on cardiovascular endpoints in high-risk patients [50].

Retinopathy

Retinopathy will eventually appear in almost all type 1 and 2 diabetic patients with vision-threatening retinal disease occurring in up to 30% of these patients [86,87]. Hyperglycemia is a major factor but there is increasing evidence for hemodynamic factors such as increased blood pressure also playing a role. In the study by the United Kingdom Prospective Diabetes Study Group (UKPDS) it was clearly demonstrated that there was a link between blood pressure and retinopathy [88]. Furthermore, in that study tight blood pressure control was associated with less retinopathy [89]. The retina has all the components of the RAS [90] and AII is a potent stimulator of a major angiogenic cytokine, vascular endothelial growth factor (VEGF), which is up-regulated in diabetes-associated proliferative retinopathy [91]. Further studies suggest that another AII-dependent growth factor, connective tissue growth factor (CTGF), which has been shown to also have angiogenic actions, may also be implicated in diabetic retinopathy. Indeed, retinal CTGF expression is attenuated by agents that interrupt the RAS [92]. Various experimental studies have reported reductions in VEGF expression in a number of retinopathy models including diabetes with ACE inhibitors and AT1 receptor antagonists [93–96]. The EURODIAB Controlled Trial of Lisinopril in Insulin-dependent Diabetes Mellitus (EUCLID) study demonstrated a reduction in the progression of human diabetic retinopathy with the ACE inhibitor, lisinopril [97]. Therefore, this potential retinoprotective action of inhibitors of the RAS is now under clinical investigation in the DIabetic REtinopathy Candesartan Trial (DIRECT) involving the use of the AT1 receptor antagonist candesartan in type 1 and 2 diabetic subjects with and without retinopathy [93].

Antihypertensive treatment and prevention of diabetes

It has been considered that thiazide diuretics and β-blockers may promote the development of type 2 diabetes mellitus. In a recent prospective study, after adjustment for age, sex, race, education, adiposity, and family history of diabetes, no increased risk for the subsequent development of diabetes was observed in thiazide-treated subjects [98]. By contrast, subjects with hypertension taking β-blockers had a 28% higher risk of subsequent diabetes. However, this adverse effect must be considered in the context of the proven benefits of β-blockers in reducing the risk of cardiovascular events including in diabetic subjects [99].

A number of studies over the past decade have suggested that ACE inhibitors may prevent or at least retard the development of diabetes, including the Heart Outcomes Prevention Evaluation (HOPE) study [73,100], the Captopril Prevention Project (CAPPP) [101,102], Australian National Blood Pressure Study (ANBP-2) [103,104], and the Studies Of Left Ventricular Dysfunction (SOLVD) trial [105]) with a reduction in new onset diabetes of between 20% to 30%. This has been further supported by findings in the ALLHAT study [82] showing that the incidence of new onset diabetes was lowest in the lisinopril group followed by the amlodipine- and chlorthalidone-treated groups. The most recent trial is the ASCOT trial [81], which demonstrated that a reduction in new-onset diabetes is not lost in combination treatments combining the CCB amlodipine with the ACE inhibitor perindopril. However, it is not surprising that the ACE inhibitor/CCB combination group was superior to the comparator group since that group included the combination of atenolol and the thiazide bendroflumethiazide, a regimen known to have particularly adverse metabolic effects.

These benefits on glucose homeostasis, seen with ACE inhibitors, have also been observed with ARBs, consistent with the major effect being via AII-dependent pathways. This needs to be considered in the context that various studies, albeit in vitro or acute clinical studies, have suggested that bradykinin may play a role in glucose tolerance [9]. The Valsartan Antihypertensive Long-term Use Evaluation (VALUE) study [106] was a very large trial that compared the CCB amlodipine to the ARB valsartan. In that study, there was a 23% reduction in the incidence of new-onset diabetes in the valsartan group, consistent with the view that the antidiabetogenic effects observed with ACE inhibitors also translate to ARBs. Similar results were obtained in the LIFE study comparing atenolol with another ARB, losartan.

A number of recently published meta-analyses including one by our own group [107,108] have suggested a potentially beneficial action of agents that interrupt the RAS, although the prevention of diabetes was not a primary endpoint in these studies. Furthermore, interpretation of the results from these studies may have been confounded by the different definitions of diabetes in the various studies and the changing criteria for the diagnosis of this condition over the past decade. Indeed, in most of these studies plasma glucose levels and assessment of glucose tolerance were not assessed adequately. The results of ongoing trials, which have been appropriately designed including the Nateglinide And Valsartan in Impaired Glucose Tolerance Outcomes Research (NAVIGATOR) [109] and the Diabetes Reduction Approaches with Ramipril and Rosiglitazone Medications (DREAM) [110] trials using valsartan and ramipril respectively are awaited to confirm the metabolic effects of RAS blockade.

The underlying mechanisms responsible for this effect of these agents on glucose homeostasis have not been fully defined but may involve effects of these inhibitors of the RAS on insulin resistance at the cellular level including inhibition of AII-mediated effects on insulin signaling or protective effects on pancreatic structure and function [111–113]. Indeed, several studies including one by our group have demonstrated in two different models of insulin resistance, the Otsuka Long-Evans Tokushima fatty rat (OLETF) [111] and the Zucker rat [113], that ACE inhibitors and AII antagonists reduce pancreatic islet fibrosis in association with reduced expression of the prosclerotic growth factors, TGF-β and CTGF, as well as reducing beta cell apoptosis and promoting beta cell proliferation.

Summary

Over the past decade there have been a large number of well-designed studies addressing the role of antihypertensive therapy in diabetic populations on a range of micro- and macrovascular endpoints. The evidence that certain antihypertensive agents such as drugs that interrupt the RAS are superior in terms of renal protection is now very convincing. We await with great anticipation the imminent findings from the DIRECT study [4,93] as to the role of RAS blockade in the prevention and retardation of diabetic retinopathy. The effects of antihypertensive treatments on macrovascular disease, left ventricular hypertrophy, and heart failure continue to be clearly shown in the diabetic population but the superiority of one class of drugs over another has not been fully elucidated. Ongoing studies such as ONTARGET [50] and the Action in Diabetes and Vascular Disease study (ADVANCE) [60] should extend our understanding as to what the target blood pressure should be in the diabetic patient and which combinations are the best not only in terms of end-organ protection but also on glucose and lipid metabolism. Indeed, one of the most exciting aspects of potential benefits of RAS blockade relates to the increasingly appreciated effects with both ACE inhibitors and ARBs on prevention and retardation of the development of type 2 diabetes. Current ongoing clinical trials will greatly assist in confirming this potential benefit although the mechanisms responsible for this metabolic advantage of such agents remain to be fully delineated. Finally, the recent identification of new components of the RAS such as the enzyme ACE2 and the putative renin receptor and the increased interest in aldosterone antagonists should provide fertile territory to not only examine new targets linked to the RAAS but potentially to design more rational treatments. These therapies aim not only to reduce diabetes-related end-organ complications, often exacerbated by hypertension, but also to attenuate or retard the progression of the insulin-resistance syndrome in which diabetes and hypertension are such important clinical manifestations.

References

[1] Cooper ME, Johnston CI. Optimizing treatment of hypertension in patients with diabetes. JAMA 2000;283(24):3177–9.
[2] Epstein M. Aldosterone receptor blockade and the role of eplerenone: evolving perspectives. Nephrol Dial Transplant 2003;18(10):1984–92.
[3] Pitt B, Williams G, Remme W, et al. The EPHESUS trial: eplerenone in patients with heart failure due to systolic dysfunction complicating acute myocardial infarction. Eplerenone Post-AMI Heart Failure Efficacy and Survival Study. Cardiovasc Drugs Ther 2001; 15(1):79–87.
[4] Chaturvedi N, Sjoelie AK, Svensson A. The DIabetic Retinopathy Candesartan Trials (DIRECT) Programme, rationale and study design. J Renin Angiotensin Aldosterone Syst 2002;3(4):255–61.
[5] Poulsen PL, Hansen KW, Mogensen CE. Ambulatory blood pressure in the transition from normo- to microalbuminuria. A longitudinal study in IDDM patients. Diabetes 1994;43: 1248–53.
[6] EDIC. Sustained effect of intensive treatment of type 1 diabetes mellitus on development and progression of diabetic nephropathy: the Epidemiology of Diabetes Interventions and Complications (EDIC) study. JAMA 2003;290(16):2159–67.
[7] Elliott MD, Kapoor A, Parker MA, et al. Improvement in hypertension in patients with diabetes mellitus after kidney/pancreas transplantation. Circulation 2001;104(5):563–9.
[8] Williams B. Insulin resistance: the shape of things to come. Lancet 1994;344:521–4.

[9] Sowers JR, Epstein M, Frohlich ED. Diabetes, hypertension, and cardiovascular disease— An update [review]. Hypertension 2001;37(4):1053–9.

[10] Eckel RH, Grundy SM, Zimmet PZ. The metabolic syndrome. Lancet 2005;365(9468): 1415–28.

[11] Isomaa B, Almgren P, Tuomi T, et al. Cardiovascular morbidity and mortality associated with the metabolic syndrome. Diabetes Care 2001;24(4):683–9.

[12] Stern N, Grosskopf I, Shapira I, et al. Risk factor clustering in hypertensive patients: impact of the reports of NCEP-II and second joint task force on coronary prevention on JNC-VI guidelines. J Intern Med 2000;248(3):203–10.

[13] Ferrannini E, Buzzigoli G, Bonadonna R, et al. Insulin resistance in essential hypertension. N Engl J Med 1987;317(6):350–7.

[14] Fukuda N, Satoh C, Hu WY, et al. Endogenous angiotensin II suppresses insulin signaling in vascular smooth muscle cells from spontaneously hypertensive rats. J Hypertens 2001; 19(9):1651–8.

[15] Vedovato M, Lepore G, Coracina A, et al. Effect of sodium intake on blood pressure and albuminuria in Type 2 diabetic patients: the role of insulin resistance. Diabetologia 2004; 47(2):300–3.

[16] Cusi K, Maezono K, Osman A, et al. Insulin resistance differentially affects the PI 3-ki-nase- and MAP kinase-mediated signaling in human muscle. J Clin Invest 2000;105(3): 311–20.

[17] Cardillo C, Nambi SS, Kilcoyne CM, et al. Insulin stimulates both endothelin and nitric oxide activity in the human forearm. Circulation 1999;100(8):820–5.

[18] Vicent D, Ilany J, Kondo T, et al. The role of endothelial insulin signaling in the regulation of vascular tone and insulin resistance. J Clin Invest 2003;111(9):1373–80.

[19] Irving RJ, Noon JP, Watt GC, et al. Activation of the endothelin system in insulin resis-tance. QJM 2001;94(6):321–6.

[20] Tooke JE. Microvascular function in human diabetes. A physiological perspective. Diabe-tes 1995;44(7):721–6.

[21] Muller-Wieland D, Kotzka J, Knebel B, et al. Metabolic syndrome and hypertension: path-ophysiology and molecular basis of insulin resistance. Basic Res Cardiol 1998;93(Suppl 2): 131–4.

[22] Cooper ME. Pathogenesis, prevention and treatment of diabetic nephropathy. Lancet 1998;352:213–9.

[23] Burns KD. Angiotensin II and its receptors in the diabetic kidney [review]. Am J Kidney Dis 2000;36(3):449–67.

[24] Anderson S, Jung FF, Ingelfinger JR. Renal renin-angiotensin system in diabetes: func-tional, immunohistochemical, and molecular biological correlations. Am J Physiol 1993; 265(4 Pt 2):F477–86.

[25] Zimpelmann J, Kumar D, Levine DZ, et al. Early diabetes mellitus stimulates proximal tubule renin mRNA expression in the rat. Kidney Int 2000;58(6):2320–30.

[26] Kelly DJ, Skinner SL, Gilbert RE, et al. Effects of endothelin or angiotensin II receptor blockade on diabetes in the transgenic (mRen-2)27 rat. Kidney Int 2000;57(5):1882–94.

[27] Taal MW, Brenner BM. Renoprotective benefits of RAS inhibition: from ACEI to angio-tensin II antagonists. Kidney Int 2000;57(5):1803–17.

[28] Taal MW, Chertow GM, Rennke HG, et al. Mechanisms underlying renoprotection during renin-angiotensin system blockade. Am J Physiol Renal Physiol 2001;280(2):F343–55.

[29] Bonnet F, Cooper ME, Kawachi H, et al. Irbesartan normalises the deficiency in glomer-ular nephrin expression in a model of diabetes and hypertension. Diabetologia 2001;44: 874–7.

[30] Hostetter TH, Rosenberg ME, Ibrahim HN, et al. Aldosterone in renal disease. Curr Opin Nephrol Hypertens 2001;10(1):105–10.

[31] Danser AH, Deinum J. Renin, prorenin and the putative (pro)renin receptor. Hypertension 2005;46(5):1069–76.

[32] Allen TJ, Cooper ME, Gilbert RE, et al. Serum total renin is increased before microalbu-
     minuria in diabetes. Kidney Int 1996;50(3):902–7.
[33] Kelly DJ, Wilkinson-Berka JL, Allen TJ, et al. A new model of diabetic nephropathy with
     progressive renal impairment in the transgenic (mRen-2)27 rat (TGR). Kidney Int 1998;
     54(2):343–52.
[34] Ichihara A, Hayashi M, Kaneshiro Y, et al. Inhibition of diabetic nephropathy by a decoy
     peptide corresponding to the "handle" region for nonproteolytic activation of prorenin.
     J Clin Invest 2004;114(8):1128–35.
[35] Nguyen G, Delarue F, Burckle C, et al. Pivotal role of the renin/prorenin receptor in angio-
     tensin II production and cellular responses to renin. J Clin Invest 2002;109(11):1417–27.
[36] Jacobsen P, Tarnow L, Carstensen B, et al. Genetic variation in the renin-angiotensin sys-
     tem and progression of diabetic nephropathy. J Am Soc Nephrol 2003;14(11):2843–50.
[37] Burrell LM, Johnston CI, Tikellis C, et al. ACE2, a new regulator of the renin-angiotensin
     system. Trends Endocrinol Metab 2004;15(4):166–9.
[38] Crackower MA, Sarao R, Oudit GY, et al. Angiotensin-converting enzyme 2 is an essential
     regulator of heart function. Nature 2002;417(6891):822–8.
[39] Tikellis C, Johnston CI, Forbes JM, et al. Characterization of renal angiotensin-converting
     enzyme 2 in diabetic nephropathy. Hypertension 2003;41(3):392–7.
[40] Li N, Zimpelmann J, Cheng K, et al. The role of angiotensin converting enzyme 2 in the
     generation of angiotensin 1–7 by rat proximal tubules. Am J Physiol Renal Physiol 2005;
     288(2):F353–62.
[41] Lewis EJ, Hunsicker LG, Bain RP, et al. The effect of angiotensin-converting-enzyme inhi-
     bition on diabetic nephropathy. The Collaborative Study Group. N Engl J Med 1993;
     329(20):1456–62.
[42] Brenner BM, Cooper ME, de Zeeuw D, et al. Effects of losartan on renal and cardiovascular
     outcomes in patients with type 2 diabetes and nephropathy. N Engl J Med 2001;345(12):
     861–9.
[43] Lewis EJ, Hunsicker LG, Clarke WR, et al. Renoprotective effect of the angiotensin-recep-
     tor antagonist irbesartan in patients with nephropathy due to type 2 diabetes. N Engl J Med
     2001;345(12):851–60.
[44] Parving HH, Lehnert H, Brochner-Mortensen J, et al. The effect of irbesartan on the devel-
     opment of diabetic nephropathy in patients with type 2 diabetes. N Engl J Med 2001;
     345(12):870–8.
[45] The ACE. Inhibitors in diabetic nephropathy trialist group: should all patients with type 1
     diabetes mellitus and microalbuminuria receive angiotensin-converting enzyme inhibitors?
     A meta-analysis of individual patient data. Ann Intern Med 2001;134(5):370–9.
[46] Allen TJ, Cao Z, Youssef S, et al. The role of angiotensin II and bradykinin in experimental
     diabetic nephropathy: functional and structural studies. Diabetes 1997;46:1612–8.
[47] Andersen S, Tarnow L, Rossing P, et al. Renoprotective effects of angiotensin II receptor
     blockade in type 1 diabetic patients with diabetic nephropathy. Kidney Int 2000;57(2):601–6.
[48] Barnett AH. The role of angiotensin II receptor antagonists in the management of diabetes.
     Blood Press 2001;10(Suppl 1):21–6.
[49] Barnett AH. Preventing renal complications in diabetic patients: the Diabetics Exposed to
     Telmisartan And enalaprIL (DETAIL) study. Acta Diabetol 2005;42(Suppl 1):S42–9.
[50] Teo K, Yusuf S, Sleight P, et al. Rationale, design, and baseline characteristics of 2 large,
     simple, randomized trials evaluating telmisartan, ramipril, and their combination in
     high-risk patients: the Ongoing Telmisartan Alone and in Combination with Ramipril
     Global Endpoint Trial/Telmisartan Randomized Assessment Study in ACE Intolerant
     Subjects with Cardiovascular Disease (ONTARGET/TRANSCEND) trials. Am Heart J
     2004;148(1):52–61.
[51] Haller H, Viberti GC, Mimran A, et al. Preventing microalbuminuria in patients with di-
     abetes: rationale and design of the Randomised Olmesartan and Diabetes Microalbuminu-
     ria Prevention (ROADMAP) study. J Hypertens 2006;24(2):403–8.

[52] Epstein M. Aldosterone and the hypertensive kidney: its emerging role as a mediator of progressive renal dysfunction: a paradigm shift. J Hypertens 2001;19(5):829–42.

[53] Rossing K, Schjoedt KJ, Smidt UM, et al. Beneficial effects of adding spironolactone to recommended antihypertensive treatment in diabetic nephropathy: a randomized, double-masked, cross-over study. Diabetes Care 2005;28(9):2106–12.

[54] Schjoedt KJ, Rossing K, Juul TR, et al. Beneficial impact of spironolactone in diabetic nephropathy. Diabetologia 2005;48(Suppl1):A6.

[55] Jacobsen PK, Rossing K, Schjoedt KJ, et al. Beneficial effects of adding spironolactone to recommended antihypertensive treatment in diabetic nephropathy. Diabetologia 2005; 48(Suppl1):A6.

[56] van den Meiracker AH, Baggen R, Boomsma F. Anti-proteinuric effect of spironolactone in type 2 diabetic nephropathy: a randomized placebo-controlled study. Diabetologia 2005; 48(Suppl1):A6–7.

[57] Epstein M, Buckalew VJ, Martinez F, et al. Antiproteinuric efficacy of eplerenone, enalapril, and eplerenone/enalapril combination therapy in diabetic hypertensives with microalbuminuria. Am J Hypertens 2002;15:24A.

[58] Jones DW, Hall JE. Seventh report of the Joint National Committee on Prevention, Detection, Evaluation, and Treatment of High Blood Pressure and evidence from new hypertension trials. Hypertension 2004;43(1):1–3.

[59] Mogensen CE, Viberti G, Halimi S, et al. Effect of low-dose perindopril/indapamide on albuminuria in diabetes: preterax in albuminuria regression: PREMIER. Hypertension 2003; 41(5):1063–71.

[60] ADVANCE–Action in Diabetes and Vascular Disease. Patient recruitment and characteristics of the study population at baseline. Diabet Med 2005;22(7):882–8.

[61] Bakris GL, Weir MR, Secic M, et al. Differential effects of calcium antagonist subclasses on markers of nephropathy progression. Kidney Int 2004;65(6):1991–2002.

[62] Bakris GL, Gaxiola E, Messerli FH, et al. Clinical outcomes in the diabetes cohort of the INternational VErapamil SR-Trandolapril study. Hypertension 2004;44(5): 637–42.

[63] Ruggenenti P, Fassi A, Ilieva AP, et al. Preventing microalbuminuria in type 2 diabetes. N Engl J Med 2004;351(19):1941–51.

[64] Mogensen CE, Neldam S, Tikkanen I, et al. Randomised controlled trial of dual blockade of renin-angiotensin system in patients with hypertension, microalbuminuria, and non-insulin dependent diabetes: the candesartan and lisinopril microalbuminuria (CALM) study. BMJ 2000;321(7274):1440–4.

[65] Rossing K, Christensen PK, Jensen BR, et al. Dual blockade of the renin-angiotensin system in diabetic nephropathy: a randomized double-blind crossover study. Diabetes Care 2002;25(1):95–100.

[66] Jacobsen P, Andersen S, Rossing K, et al. Dual blockade of the renin-angiotensin system in type 1 patients with diabetic nephropathy. Nephrol Dial Transplant 2002;17(6): 1019–24.

[67] Jacobsen P, Andersen S, Jensen BR, et al. Additive effect of ACE inhibition and angiotensin II receptor blockade in type I diabetic patients with diabetic nephropathy. J Am Soc Nephrol 2003;14(4):992–9.

[68] Jacobsen P, Andersen S, Rossing K, et al. Dual blockade of the renin-angiotensin system versus maximal recommended dose of ACE inhibition in diabetic nephropathy. Kidney Int 2003;63(5):1874–80.

[69] Rossing K, Jacobsen P, Pietraszek L, et al. Renoprotective effects of adding angiotensin II receptor blocker to maximal recommended doses of ACE inhibitor in diabetic nephropathy: a randomized double-blind crossover trial. Diabetes Care 2003;26(8):2268–74.

[70] Sengul AM, Altuntas Y, Kurklu A, et al. Beneficial effect of lisinopril plus telmisartan in patients with type 2 diabetes, microalbuminuria and hypertension. Diabetes Res Clin Pract 2006;71(2):210–9.

[71] Andersen NH, Poulsen PL, Knudsen ST, et al. Long-term dual blockade with candesartan and lisinopril in hypertensive patients with diabetes: the CALM II study. Diabetes Care 2005;28(2):273–7.

[72] Rossing K, Schjoedt KJ, Jensen BR, et al. Enhanced renoprotective effects of ultrahigh doses of irbesartan in patients with type 2 diabetes and microalbuminuria. Kidney Int 2005;68(3):1190–8.

[73] Gerstein HC, Yusuf S, Mann JFE, et al. Effects of ramipril on cardiovascular and microvascular outcomes in people with diabetes mellitus: results of the HOPE study and MICRO-HOPE substudy. Lancet 2000;355(9200):253–9.

[74] Azizi M, Menard J. Combined blockade of the renin-angiotensin system with angiotensin-converting enzyme inhibitors and angiotensin II type 1 receptor antagonists. Circulation 2004;109(21):2492–9.

[75] Agmon Y, Khandheria BK, Meissner I, et al. Independent association of high blood pressure and aortic atherosclerosis—A population-based study. Circulation 2000;102(17): 2087–93.

[76] Kuperstein R, Hanly P, Niroumand M, et al. The importance of age and obesity on the relation between diabetes and left ventricular mass. J Am Coll Cardiol 2001;37(7):1957–62.

[77] Dwyer EM, Asif M, Ippolito T, et al. Role of hypertension, diabetes, obesity, and race in the development of symptomatic myocardial dysfunction in a predominantly minority population with normal coronary arteries. Am Heart J 2000;139(2 Part 1):297–304.

[78] Dawson A, Morris AD, Struthers AD. The epidemiology of left ventricular hypertrophy in type 2 diabetes mellitus. Diabetologia 2005;48(10):1971–9.

[79] Bella JN, Devereux RB, Roman MJ, et al. Separate and joint effects of systemic hypertension and diabetes mellitus on left ventricular structure and function in American Indians (the strong heart study). Am J Cardiol 2001;87(11):1260–5.

[80] Boner G, Cooper ME, McCarroll K, et al. Adverse effects of left ventricular hypertrophy in the reduction of endpoints in NIDDM with the angiotensin II antagonist losartan (RENAAL) study. Diabetologia 2005;48(10):1980–7.

[81] Dahlof B, Sever PS, Poulter NR, et al. Prevention of cardiovascular events with an antihypertensive regimen of amlodipine adding perindopril as required versus atenolol adding bendroflumethiazide as required, in the Anglo-Scandinavian Cardiac Outcomes Trial-Blood Pressure Lowering Arm (ASCOT-BPLA): a multicentre randomised controlled trial. Lancet 2005;366(9489):895–906.

[82] The Antihypertensive and Lipid-Lowering Treatment to Prevent Heart Attack Trial (ALLHAT). Major outcomes in high-risk hypertensive patients randomized to angiotensin-converting enzyme inhibitor or calcium channel blocker vs diuretic. JAMA 2002;288(23): 2981–97.

[83] Whelton PK, Barzilay J, Cushman WC, et al. Clinical outcomes in antihypertensive treatment of type 2 diabetes, impaired fasting glucose concentration, and normoglycemia: Antihypertensive and Lipid-Lowering Treatment to Prevent Heart Attack Trial (ALLHAT). Arch Intern Med 2005;165(12):1401–9.

[84] Poulter NR, Wedel H, Dahlof B, et al. Role of blood pressure and other variables in the differential cardiovascular event rates noted in the Anglo-Scandinavian Cardiac Outcomes Trial-Blood Pressure Lowering Arm (ASCOT-BPLA). Lancet 2005;366(9489):907–13.

[85] Frustaci A, Kajstura J, Chimenti C, et al. Myocardial cell death in human diabetes. Circ Res 2000;87(12):1123–32.

[86] Wong TY, Mitchell P. Hypertensive retinopathy. N Engl J Med 2004;351(22):2310–7.

[87] Wong TY, Duncan BB, Golden SH, et al. Associations between the metabolic syndrome and retinal microvascular signs: the Atherosclerosis Risk In Communities study. Invest Ophthalmol Vis Sci 2004;45(9):2949–54.

[88] Stratton IM, Kohner EM, Aldington SJ, et al. UKPDS 50: risk factors for incidence and progression of retinopathy in Type II diabetes over 6 years from diagnosis. Diabetologia 2001;44(2):156–63.

[89] UK Prospective Diabetes Study Group. Tight blood pressure control and risk of macrovascular and microvascular complications in type 2 diabetes: UKPDS 38. BMJ 1998; 317(7160):703–13.

[90] Wagner J, Danser AHJ, Derkx FHM, et al. Demonstration of renin mrna, angiotensinogen mrna, and angiotensin converting enzyme mrna expression in the human eye—evidence for an intraocular renin-angiotensin system. Br J Ophthalmol 1996;80(2):159–63.

[91] Aiello LP, Avery RL, Arrigg PG, et al. Vascular endothelial growth factor in ocular fluid of patients with diabetic retinopathy and other retinal disorders. N Engl J Med 1994;331(22): 1480–7.

[92] Tikellis C, Cooper ME, Twigg SM, et al. Connective tissue growth factor is up-regulated in the diabetic retina: amelioration by angiotensin-converting enzyme inhibition. Endocrinology 2004;145(2):860–6.

[93] Sjølie A, Porta M, Parving HH, et al. The DIabetic REtinopathy Candesartan Trial (DIRECT) Programme. J Renin Angiotensin Aldosterone Syst 2005;6(1):25–32.

[94] Nagisa Y, Shintani A, Nakagawa S. The angiotensin II receptor antagonist candesartan cilexetil (TCV-116) ameliorates retinal disorders in rats. Diabetologia 2001;44(7): 883–8.

[95] Gilbert RE, Kelly DJ, Cox AJ, et al. Angiotensin converting enzyme inhibition reduces retinal overexpression of vascular endothelial growth factor and hyperpermeability in experimental diabetes. Diabetologia 2000;43(11):1360–7.

[96] Moravski CJ, Kelly DJ, Cooper ME, et al. Retinal neovascularization is prevented by blockade of the renin-angiotensin system. Hypertension 2000;36(6):1099–104.

[97] Chaturvedi N, Sjolie A-K, Stephenson JM, et al. Effect of lisinopril on progression of retinopathy in people with type 1 diabetes. Lancet 1998;351:28–31.

[98] Gress TW, Nieto FJ, Shahar E, et al. Hypertension and antihypertensive therapy as risk factors for type 2 diabetes mellitus. N Engl J Med 2000;342(13):905–12.

[99] Gilbert RE, Cooper ME, Krum H. Drug administration in patients with diabetes mellitus. Safety considerations. Drug Saf 1998;18(6):441–55.

[100] Yusuf S, Gerstein H, Hoogwerf B, et al. Ramipril and the development of diabetes. JAMA 2001;286(15):1882–5.

[101] Hansson L, Lindholm LH, Niskanen L, et al. Effect of angiotensin-converting-enzyme inhibition compared with conventional therapy on cardiovascular morbidity and mortality in hypertension: the Captopril Prevention Project (CAPPP) randomised trial. Lancet 1999; 353(9153):611–6.

[102] Niklason A, Hedner T, Niskanen L, et al. Development of diabetes is retarded by ACE inhibition in hypertensive patients–a subanalysis of the Captopril Prevention Project (CAPPP). J Hypertens 2004;22(3):645–52.

[103] Wing LM, Reid CM, Ryan P, et al. A comparison of outcomes with angiotensin-converting–enzyme inhibitors and diuretics for hypertension in the elderly. N Engl J Med 2003;348(7):583–92.

[104] Reid CM, Jonston CI, Ryan P, et al. Diabetes and cardiovascular outcomes in elderly subjects treated with ACE-inhibitors or diuretics: findings from the 2nd Australian National Blood Pressure Study [abstract]. Am J Hypertens 2003;16 (5[Suppl]):A11.

[105] Vermes E, Ducharme A, Bourassa MG, et al. Enalapril reduces the incidence of diabetes in patients with chronic heart failure: insight from the Studies Of Left Ventricular Dysfunction (SOLVD). Circulation 2003;107(9):1291–6.

[106] Julius S, Kjeldsen SE, Weber M, et al. Outcomes in hypertensive patients at high cardiovascular risk treated with regimens based on valsartan or amlodipine: the VALUE randomised trial. Lancet 2004;363(9426):2022–31.

[107] Jandeleit-Dahm KA, Tikellis C, Reid CM, et al. Why blockade of the renin-angiotensin system reduces the incidence of new-onset diabetes. J Hypertens 2005;23(3):463–73.

[108] Elliott WJ. Differential effects of antihypertensive drugs on new-onset diabetes? Curr Hypertens Rep 2005;7(4):249–56.

[109] Chiasson JL, Brindisi MC, Rabasa-Lhoret R. The prevention of type 2 diabetes: what is the evidence? Minerva Endocrinol 2005;30(3):179–91.

[110] Gerstein HC, Yusuf S, Holman R, et al. Rationale, design and recruitment characteristics of a large, simple international trial of diabetes prevention: the DREAM trial. Diabetologia 2004;47(9):1519–27.

[111] Ko SH, Kwon HS, Kim SR, et al. Ramipril treatment suppresses islet fibrosis in Otsuka Long-Evans Tokushima fatty rats. Biochem Biophys Res Commun 2004;316(1):114–22.

[112] Tikellis C, Cooper ME, Thomas MC. Role of the renin-angiotensin system in the endocrine pancreas: implications for the development of diabetes. Int J Biochem Cell Biol 2006;38: 737–51.

[113] Tikellis C, Wookey PJ, Candido R, et al. Improved islet morphology after blockade of the renin-angiotensin system in the ZDF rat. Diabetes 2004;53(4):989–97.

ELSEVIER
SAUNDERS

Endocrinol Metab Clin N Am
35 (2006) 491–510

ENDOCRINOLOGY
AND METABOLISM
CLINICS
OF NORTH AMERICA

Diabetic Dyslipidemia

Tina J. Chahil, MD, Henry N. Ginsberg, MD*

*Department of Medicine, College of Physicians and Surgeons of Columbia University,
PH 10-305, 630 West 168th Street, New York, NY 10032, USA*

Diabetic dyslipidemia and cardiovascular disease

Evidence has established a definitive link between diabetes mellitus and the risk of cardiovascular disease. Worldwide and United States estimates attribute 52% to 65% of deaths among diabetics to cardiovascular causes, particularly ischemic heart disease and cerebrovascular events [1–3]. The presence of diabetes confers a twofold to fourfold increase in the risk of coronary artery disease, and similar increases in the risk of stroke and rates of peripheral arterial disease [3–5]. In the absence of established heart disease, older diabetics with longstanding disease have as high a risk for fatal cardiovascular events as nondiabetics with previously diagnosed coronary heart disease (CHD) [6–8]. In the setting of previous heart disease, diabetes has been associated consistently with greater risk for short-term and long-term cardiovascular morbidity and mortality [9]. The magnification of cardiovascular risk associated with diabetes is even more striking in women [10]. Diabetes appears to negate the protective effect against cardiovascular disease afforded women in their premenopausal years, possibly because diabetes exerts a greater negative impact in women, relative to men, on multiple cardiovascular risk factors, such as waist-to-hip ratio, high-density lipoprotein (HDL) and low-density lipoprotein (LDL) cholesterol levels, and plasma apolipoprotein A-1 (apoA-I) and apolipoprotein B (apoB) concentrations [6,8,11–13].

Although the increased risk for cardiovascular disease among patients who have diabetes is multifactorial in nature, much of the excess risk can be attributed to diabetic dyslipidemia, which is characterized by increased levels of very low-density lipoprotein (VLDL) triglycerides (TG) and apoB, reduced levels of HDL cholesterol and its major structural protein, apoA-I, and a predominance of small, cholesteryl ester–poor LDL. The predominance of cholesteryl

---

* Corresponding author.
E-mail address: hng1@columbia.edu (H.N. Ginsberg).

0889-8529/06/$ - see front matter © 2006 Elsevier Inc. All rights reserved.
doi:10.1016/j.ecl.2006.06.002

ester–poor LDL results in increased numbers of LDL particles (as denoted by a high total apoB concentration), even when LDL cholesterol levels are normal. In addition, abnormalities in postprandial lipid metabolism parallel those present during the fasting state. Because of the central role of insulin resistance in the pathophysiology of the dyslipidemia seen in diabetes, abnormalities of plasma lipids and lipoproteins are present long before the development of overt hyperglycemia, underscoring their significant contribution to the risk of macrovascular disease [14–16].

Introduction to normal lipoprotein metabolism

Before describing in detail the pathophysiology of the characteristic diabetic dyslipidemia, some basic definitions and facts of normal lipoprotein metabolism need to be reviewed. Lipoproteins are macromolecular complexes composed of various amounts of TG, free and esterified cholesterol, phospholipids, and proteins. They function primarily in the transport of the very hydrophobic TG and cholesteryl esters between either the intestine or the liver and the peripheral tissues, particularly muscle and adipose tissue. The phospholipids on the surface of all lipoproteins are amphipathic, allowing them to functionally solubilize the very hydrophobic core lipids as they traverse the aqueous plasma. Although lipoproteins exist as a continuum in terms of size, density, and lipid composition, they can, based on accumulation of particles in certain density ranges, be divided into five major classes: chylomicrons; VLDL; intermediate-density lipoprotein (IDL) (also referred to as VLDL remnants in this review); LDL; and HDL. These lipoprotein classes differ in the core lipids they carry, and in their surface proteins, called apolipoproteins. Apolipoproteins are important modulators of lipoprotein function because they act as ligands for various lipoprotein receptors and can inhibit or activate enzymes that are important for lipoprotein metabolism (Table 1).

Two key apolipoproteins, which characterize three series of lipoproteins, are apoA-I and apoB. ApoB is present in a full-length form made in the liver (apoB100) and a truncated form made in the intestine (apoB48). ApoB48 defines intestinally derived chylomicrons and their remnants, whereas apoB100 defines liver-derived VLDL, IDL, and LDL. Each of these lipoproteins has one apoB molecule. Thus, the concentration of apoB is a good surrogate for the number of apoB-lipoproteins present in the circulation. This is important because all apoB-lipoproteins except nascent chylomicrons have the potential to initiate atherogenesis because they can penetrate the artery wall, enter the subendothelial space, and be oxidatively modified. ApoA-I, made in the small intestine and liver, defines the series of HDL. ApoA-I lipoproteins are antiatherogenic. Several reasons for HDL's protective effects have been proposed, including anti-inflammatory and antioxidant activities, and the ability to inhibit vascular smooth muscle cell migration. However, it is the role of HDL in reverse cholesterol transport (RCT) that is generally accepted as its most important antiatherogenic

Table 1
Characteristics of the major apolipoproteins

Apolipoprotein	M	Lipoproteins	Metabolic functions
apoA-I	28,016	HDL, chylomicrons	Structural component of HDL; LCAT activator
apoA-II	17,414	HDL, chylomicrons	Unknown
apoA-IV	46, 465	HDL, chylomicrons	Unknown; possibly facilitates transfer of apos between HDL and chylomicrons
apoA-V	39,000	HDL	Associated with lower TG levels; facilitates LpL
apoB-48	264,000	Chylomicrons	Necessary for assembly and secretion of chylomicrons from the small intestine
apoB-100	514,000	VLDL, IDL, LDL	Necessary for secretion of VLDL from liver structural protein of VLDL, IDL and LDL; ligand for the LDL receptor
apoC-I	6,630	Chylomicrons, VLDL, IDL, HDL	May inhibit hepatic uptake of chylomicrons and VLDL remnants
apoC-II	8,900	Chylomicrons, VLDL, IDL, HDL	Activator of LpL
apoC-III	8,800	Chylomicrons, VLDL, IDL, HDL	Inhibitor of lipoprotein lipase and of uptake of chylomicron and VLDL remnant by the liver
apoE	34,145	Chylomicrons, VLDL, IDL, HDL	Ligand for binding of several lipoproteins to the LDL receptor, LRP and proteoglycans
apo(a)	250,000– 800,000	Lp(a)	Composed of LDL apoB linked covalently to apo(a); function unknown but is an independent predictor of CAD

Abbreviations: CAD, coronary artery disease; LCAT, lecithin cholesterol acyltransferase; Lp(a), lipoprotein(a); LpL, lipoprotein lipase; M, molecular mass.

function. RCT is the process whereby organs and cells, including macrophages in atherosclerotic lesions, unload cholesterol onto lipid-poor subclasses of HDL, which can then transport the sterol to the liver for eventual excretion in the bile.

Type 1 diabetes and dyslipidemia

Although most of the remaining discussion focuses on the many abnormalities in lipoprotein metabolism that occur in patients who have type 2 diabetes, the authors review this issue briefly in individuals with type 1 diabetes. Marked elevations in the levels of TG-rich lipoproteins, including both chylomicrons and VLDL, can be seen in poorly controlled type 1 diabetics because of a reduction in the activity of lipoprotein lipase (LpL), an insulin-regulated enzyme synthesized in adipose tissue and muscle that hydrolyzes TG in the core of chylomicrons and VLDL. Chylomicron and VLDL remnant removal may also be defective in the setting of insulin deficiency, because of the role of insulin in the synthesis and maturation of proteoglycans, carbohydrate-rich proteins that allow remnants to associate with hepatocyte plasma membranes, thereby facilitating their uptake [17]. When TG-rich lipoproteins are increased in patients who have type I diabetes, increased exchange of HDL and LDL cholesteryl esters for TG in chylomicrons and VLDL can reduce HDL levels and generate small, dense LDL. These exchanges, which are mediated by a plasma protein called cholesteryl ester transfer protein (CETP), are discussed in more detail later in this article. Absolute levels of LDL cholesterol and apoB100 (as a marker of the number of LDL particles) can be increased in patients who have type 1 diabetes when there is significant insulin deficiency, because LDL receptor expression is regulated, in part, by insulin. In contrast, patients who have well-controlled type 1 diabetes have serum lipid and lipoprotein levels that are the same as, or "better than," those of their nondiabetic counterparts. However, even when plasma lipid and lipoprotein levels are normal in patients who have type 1 diabetes, the apoB-lipoproteins are cholesteryl ester–enriched and potentially more atherogenic. Finally, it is possible for individuals with type 1 diabetes to also inherit insulin resistance and, if they become obese, present with a dyslipidemia that resembles the characteristic abnormalities seen in patients who have type 2 diabetes.

Type 2 diabetes and dyslipidemia

The typical dyslipidemia of type 2 diabetes is characterized by several quantitative and qualitative lipoprotein abnormalities. The most common cluster of lipid abnormalities among patients who have type 2 diabetes is the combination of elevations of both fasting and postprandial TG levels, low HDL cholesterol levels, and an increase in small, dense LDL particles. Plasma LDL cholesterol levels are generally similar between diabetics and nondiabetics, although in some studies, women with type 2 diabetes may have a modest increase in LDL cholesterol concentrations. Numerous clinical trials and observational studies have demonstrated a propensity for this pattern of dyslipidemia in diabetics (Table 2). Some studies have suggested that the predominance of smaller, cholesteryl ester–depleted LDL particles may impart a greater atherogenic risk to patients who have diabetes [18,19]. However, this view is not accepted by all workers in the field [20]. Later in this article, the authors describe the pathophysiologic mechanisms underlying each component of the diabetic dyslipidemia.

Diabetic dyslipidemia: chylomicron metabolism

Normal lipoprotein metabolism can be divided into postprandial and fasting periods. Following digestion of dietary nutrients, cells of the small

Table 2
Phenotype of the diabetic dyslipidemia compared to nondiabetic men and women

	Nondiabetic men and women	Diabetic women	Diabetic men
TC	1.00	1.00–1.09	0.96–1.04
HDL	1.00	0.74–0.86	0.87–0.92
LDL	1.00	0.95–1.01	0.90–0.96
TG	1.00	1.49–2.89	1.27–1.52

All lipid values for diabetics are normalized to those of nondiabetics of the same gender.
Abbreviation: TC, total cholesterol.
Data from Ref. 12, 13, 67, 68 (LDL data from Ref. 12, 68).

intestine absorb fatty acids (FA) and cholesterol from the diet and incorporate them, as TG and cholesteryl esters, respectively, into chylomicrons, which are secreted into the lymph. Because we eat grams of TG and only milligrams of cholesterol, chylomicrons are about 95% TG by weight. ApoB48 is required for the assembly and secretion of chylomicrons by the small intestine; it appears that, as is the case for apoB100, apoB48 is constitutively synthesized and degraded unless the influx of core lipids after a meal targets the apolipoprotein for secretion on a chylomicron. Such targeting requires not only the arrival of core lipid components, but also the activity of microsomal triglyceride transfer protein (MTP), which mediates movement of lipids onto apoB. Recent studies indicate that, like apoB100 and VLDL assembly (see below), the association of apoB48 with dietary lipids to form chylomicrons is dysregulated in the presence of insulin resistance; increased apoB48 secretion has been demonstrated in the insulin-resistant, sucrose-fed hamster [21]. It is not clear, however, if this happens in humans.

As they travel through the lymph and subsequently enter the circulation by way of the thoracic duct, chylomicrons acquire other apolipoproteins, including apoC-I, apoC-II, apoC-III, apoE, and apoA-V. ApoC-II is a required activator of LpL, the enzyme in adipose tissue and muscle that hydrolyzes (lipolyzes) chylomicron TG. ApoA-V, a recently identified apolipoprotein, appears to facilitate this process [22]. In contrast, apoC-III inhibits LpL-mediated lipolysis. In the capillary beds of fat (especially in the fed state) and muscle, the chylomicrons interact with LpL, which is synthesized and secreted from those tissues and is bound to the surface of capillary endothelial cells. ApoB48 plays a role in this interaction, which results in lipolysis of the core TG and the release of FA. Adipocytes absorb FA that have been released during lipolysis and reincorporate them into TG for storage; acylation-stimulating protein, which is made in adipocytes, appears to assist in the trapping of FA in these cells [23]. In muscle, FA from chylomicrons can be used as a source of energy. Indeed, the balance of LpL activity between fat and muscle is determined by the energy status and needs of the organism. LpL is regulated by insulin at several levels, including gene expression, protein synthesis, and secretion, and LpL is reduced modestly in insulin-resistant individuals with type 2 diabetes [24]. Studies in cell culture systems and in rodents suggest that apoC-III gene expression is regulated by insulin, possibly by the transcription factor, FOXO-1 [25], with increased apoC-III production in insulin-deficient or resistant states. Recent evidence from studies in humans indicates that individuals with insulin resistance also have overproduction of both apoC-III and VLDL apoB100 [26]. If apoC-III synthesis is increased in humans with insulin resistance, LpL action could be impaired. No studies indicate dysregulation of either apoC-II, of which very little is required for normal activation of LpL, or apoA-V in subjects with diabetes, although recent studies indicate that apoA-V gene expression is regulated, at least in part, by insulin [27]. Additionally, increased secretion of VLDL, which is characteristic of the insulin-resistant state (see below), leads to increased levels of VLDL TG that compete with chylomicrons for LpL-mediated lipolysis [28,29].

Chylomicron remnants, which are the products of lipolysis, are relatively depleted in apoC-apolipoproteins and enriched in apoE. Remnants are removed from the circulation by the liver by way of their interaction with various complexes, including the LDL receptor, the LDL receptor-related protein (LRP), hepatic lipase (HL), and cell-surface proteoglycans. ApoE plays a critical role in facilitating these interactions, whereas all of the apoC-lipoproteins can inhibit hepatic removal of the chylomicron remnant [30]. The apoE isoform pattern of any individual with diabetes can impact on chylomicron removal; apoE2, in particular, has defective binding to the LDL receptors. LDL receptors themselves are highly regulated at the gene expression level, in part by insulin. Studies of humans suggest that severe diabetes, with significant relative or absolute insulin deficiency, is accompanied by decreased clearance of LDL [31]; whether this extends to chylomicron remnant clearance is unknown. The synthesis and maturation of cell-surface proteoglycans, carbohydrate-rich proteins that allow remnants to associate with hepatocyte plasma membranes, may be defective when insulin action is reduced significantly [17]. HL, which hydrolyzes chylomicron remnant and VLDL remnant TG, has also been implicated in remnant removal [32]. Therefore, deficiency of HL might be associated with reduced remnant clearance. However, HL is elevated in individuals with insulin resistance with or without diabetes [13]. Several studies have demonstrated an association between postprandial hyperlipidemia and the presence of CHD in nondiabetics [33]. This association has not been demonstrated in subjects with type 2 diabetes, possibly because all insulin-resistant individuals have postprandial hyperlipidemia.

Diabetic dyslipidemia: assembly and secretion of very low-density lipoprotein

In the fasting state and, to a lesser degree, during the postprandial period, the liver can assemble and secrete VLDL. Like chylomicrons, VLDL are mainly TG-carrying lipoproteins, although TG make up only about 80% of the weight of VLDL. The TG that are packaged into the VLDL core are derived from several sources: FA taken up directly from the circulation; FA released from chylomicron remnants or VLDL remnants (see below) after their uptake and hydrolysis in lysosomes; or FA derived from de novo synthesis by way of hepatic lipogenesis. The sources of cholesteryl esters and free cholesterol in secreted VLDL are less well defined: chylomicron or VLDL remnant uptake, and LDL uptake, with delivery of their cholesterol to a secretory pool, are likely sources, as is endogenously synthesized cholesterol.

ApoB100 is synthesized in hepatocytes and is required for VLDL assembly and secretion. ApoB100 is the major structural protein of VLDL, IDL and LDL, and is an important ligand for the LDL receptor. Evidence from a number of laboratories studying cultured liver cells, primary hepatocytes, and whole livers indicates that apoB100 is synthesized at a relatively constant rate, with secretion of apoB100 regulated posttranscriptionally by the availability of its core lipids, TG, and cholesteryl esters [34]. Degradation of apoB100 (as well as apoB48; see above) occurs both cotranslationally and posttranslationally. In the former instance, inadequate core lipid availability leads to cotranslational exposure of apoB to the cytosolic side of the endoplasmic reticulum (ER), where it is ubiquitinylated and targeted to the proteasome for degradation [35]. Posttranslational degradation of apoB100 occurs by way of several pathways, some of which are in the ER and some post-ER [36]. As in the intestine, MTP plays a crucial role here as well: normal MTP activity is required for VLDL assembly and apoB100 secretion. Overproduction of VLDL, with increased secretion of both TG and apoB100, seems to be the central, and most important, cause of increased plasma VLDL levels in patients who have insulin resistance and type 2 diabetes mellitus [37]. This results from the targeting of apB100 away from degradation and to lipoprotein assembly. Increases in the three main sources of TG for VLDL assembly (ie, FA flux from adipose tissue to the liver; hepatic uptake of TG-enriched VLDL and chylomicron remnants; and de novo lipogenesis) are linked to the increased assembly and secretion of VLDL from the liver (Fig. 1). Whether alterations in hepatic cholesterol metabolism stimulate VLDL secretion in type 2 diabetes is not known. Additionally, MTP is increased in some, but not all, animal models of insulin resistance and increased VLDL secretion.

It has been known for more than 30 years that increased FA levels in blood and increased FA flux to the liver occur in humans with insulin resistance, with and without type 2 diabetes mellitus. It is also known that plasma albumin-bound FA are a source of VLDL TG [38]. Acutely raising plasma FA levels can increase VLDL secretion in normal individuals [39] and in rodents [40]. In the rodent study, conducted in the authors' laboratory, very small quantities of FA were required to stimulate apoB secretion, and this increase in apoB secretion was not accompanied by increases in TG secretion. This finding suggests that FA might act both as a stimulus for TG

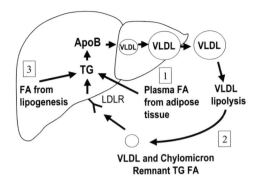

Fig. 1. The three major sources of hepatic TG, the main substrate regulating VLDL apoB secretion, are FA, which are albumin-bound and derived mainly from lipolysis of triglycerides in adipose tissue; chylomicron and VLDL remnant TG FA that are delivered to the hepatocytes by endocytosis, mainly by way of the LDL receptor (LDLR); and FA that are synthesized by de novo hepatic lipogenesis. In insulin resistance and type 2 diabetes (1), FA flux through the plasma to the liver is increased (2); peripheral removal (by lipolysis) of chylomicron and VLDL TG is reduced, leaving TG-enriched remnants for hepatic uptake (3); and de novo hepatic lipogenesis is increased. All these sources of TG may contribute to the increased VLDL secretion present in individuals with insulin resistance.

synthesis, thereby driving assembly of VLDL, and as a "signal" for apoB assembly, which is, at least partly, independent of core lipid availability.

Postprandial hyperlipidemia is common in insulin-resistant individuals, probably because of a modest reduction in LpL-mediated lipolysis of nascent chylomicrons. This abnormality is associated almost certainly with hepatic uptake of chylomicron remnants that contain more TG than do remnants in people without insulin resistance. The same problem with lipolysis occurs with VLDL; that is, TG-enriched VLDL remnants accumulate in people with insulin resistance. Uptake of these TG-enriched remnants will stimulate VLDL assembly and secretion as the liver attempts to maintain homeostasis regarding its FA acid and TG content. This phenomenon has been demonstrated in cultured liver cells [41], rodents [40] and humans [42].

The third source of TG for assembly and secretion with apoB100 is de novo hepatic lipogenesis. Several recent papers have shown that lipogenesis contributes significantly to VLDL TG, and is increased in individuals with obesity and insulin resistance [43,44]. Goldstein, Brown, and colleagues [45], defined in detail the regulation of hepatic lipogenesis by the sterol response element–binding protein 1-c (SREBP-1c). Their work indicated that hepatic SREBP-1c gene expression was regulated by insulin through another transcription factor, the liver-x-receptor. In hyperinsulinemic ob/ob mice, SREBP-1c gene expression was increased, despite resistance to insulin's actions on the hepatic carbohydrate metabolism [46].

In the authors' recent studies (unpublished), they have found that lipogenesis is increased in the apoB/BATless mouse, a model of moderate obesity, insulin resistance and increased VLDL secretion [47]. However, neither

SREBP1-c gene expression nor generation of the transcriptionally active form of the protein was altered. On the other hand, the expression and activity of the peroxisome proliferator-activated receptor gamma (PPARγ) was increased in the livers of apoB/BATless mice. This finding, together with published data indicating an important role for PPARγ in hepatic lipogenesis in other mouse models of obesity and insulin resistance, has intriguing clinical implications for the treatment of hepatic steatosis.

Insulin not only stimulates lipogenesis, but also plays a key role in determining whether apoB100 is targeted for secretion or degradation [48]. Insulin, acting by way of a P-I-3 kinase–associated pathway, can target apoB100 for degradation. This degradation is posttranslational and probably occurs post-ER. Recent studies suggest that stimulation of apoB100 degradation by insulin may be linked to high levels of oxidant stress in insulin-treated hepatocytes [49]. Decreased secretion of both VLDL TG and apoB100 has been demonstrated in normal subjects treated with large quantities of insulin and glucose (euglycemic clamps) [50]. The effects of insulin on apoB degradation appear to diminish significantly if insulin resistance is present; this is true in cultured cells, whole animals, and humans [50,51]. A potentially important and clinically relevant extension of the aforementioned finding relates to the increasing prevalence of fatty livers in people with obesity and insulin resistance, with or without type 2 diabetes. Although such individuals seem to be able to increase VLDL secretion as they attempt to maintain hepatic lipid homeostasis in the face of increased sources of TG, some cannot keep up and, as a result, TG accumulate in their hepatocytes. It is possible that the relative degrees of both insulin resistance and hyperinsulinemia determine whether a fatty liver will develop in any individual. Severe insulin resistance means that there will be enough apoB100 (because of reduced insulin-mediated degradation) to unload the TG by way of VLDL secretion, despite increased uptake of albumin-bound FA and TG-containing remnants, and regardless of the level of lipogenesis. Moderate insulin resistance, combined with adequate insulin signaling in the insulin-mediated apoB100 degradation pathway, allows TG to accumulate and a fatty liver to develop (Fig. 2). This hypothesis requires further investigation.

Diabetic dyslipidemia: very low-density lipoprotein catabolism

VLDL are secreted with some of the other apolipoproteins and acquire additional quantities of them once in the plasma. As VLDL circulate, hydrolysis of their TG component by LpL produces smaller and denser particles. ApoC-II, apoC-III, and apoA-V play regulatory roles at this step of VLDL catabolism, just as they do in chylomicron catabolism. Modest decreases in LpL that may exist in patients who have type 2 diabetes, ogether with increased production of apoC-III associated with insulin resistance, can lead to defective lipolysis. VLDL and chylomicrons can compete for the same LpL-mediated pathway for TG removal from the circulation; postprandial

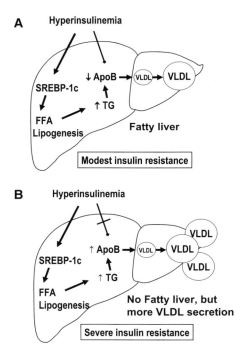

Fig. 2. Insulin regulates the balance between VLDL secretion and hepatic steatosis by stimulating de novo hepatic lipogenesis and the degradation of apoB. Hepatic insulin resistance does not seem to affect lipogenesis, but does impair insulin-mediated apoB degradation. Therefore, if plasma hyperinsulinemia is accompanied by modest hepatic insulin resistance (*A*), then lipogenesis will be increased, but so will apoB degradation, leading to the development of hepatic steatosis. However, if plasma hyperinsulinemia is paralleled by severe hepatic insulin resistance (*B*), then lipogenesis will still be increased, but apoB degradation will be low and more VLDL will be secreted, reducing the risk for steatosis. This relationship between lipogenesis and apoB degradation (both of which are regulated by insulin) will be modulated by FA taken up from the plasma by the liver, and by the TG content of remnants returning to the liver.

hyperlipidemia will, therefore, lead to inefficient VLDL TG clearance. Once adequate lipolysis has occurred, IDL, also called VLDL remnants, are generated. These lipoproteins can either be taken up by the liver by way of pathways similar to those that remove chylomicrons remnants, or undergo further removal of TG by the action of HL, resulting in the formation of LDL particles. Again, the apoC-apolipoproteins and apoE play important roles in VLDL remnant removal by the liver. Despite increased levels of apoC-III and the potential for defects in proteoglycan synthesis, the proportion of VLDL remnants that are removed by the liver (rather than being converted to LDL) is usually increased in patients who have insulin resistance. Nevertheless, the combination of increased hepatic secretion of both VLDL and TG-depleted, LDL-density apoB100-lipoproteins results in increased production of LDL in most patients who have type 2 diabetes.

Diabetic dyslipidemia: generation of small, dense low-density lipoprotein

LDL particles are composed almost exclusively of cholesteryl esters in the core and have essentially only apoB100 on the surface. Most LDL are cleared from the plasma through their interaction with the LDL receptor; about 50% of LDL are removed by the liver. In people with insulin resistance and type 2 diabetes mellitus, regulation of plasma levels of LDL, like that of its precursor, VLDL, is complex. A common characteristic of the diabetic dyslipidemia is the presence of dense, cholesteryl ester–depleted, TG-enriched LDL, a profile called pattern B [52]. The origin of small, dense LDL in insulin resistance is complex. To a large degree, they are generated by the action of CETP. This protein, which is associated with plasma lipoproteins, particularly HDL, can mediate the exchange of VLDL (or chylomicron) TG for LDL cholesteryl esters, thereby creating a TG-enriched, cholesteryl ester–depleted LDL particle. The TG in LDL can then be lipolyzed by LpL or HL, generating small, dense LDL. However, the finding that small dense LDL are present in insulin-resistant/type 2 diabetic patients, even when they have relatively normal TG levels, suggests that other factors are at play. One factor is HL, which is increased in insulin resistance, and therefore can hydrolyze TG in LDL more effectively. Higher levels of blood FA, present in individuals with diabetic dyslipidemia, have also been shown to stimulate exchange of cholesteryl esters and TG between LDL (or HDL; see below) and VLDL. Another possible factor is that even when fasting TG levels are normal, diabetics have elevated postprandial levels of chylomicrons and VLDL. Because we are actually in the postprandial state most of the time, small, dense LDL may, therefore, be indicative of significant postprandial hyperlipidemia. Finally, the type of VLDL originally assembled and secreted into the plasma may be important. Patients who have diabetes tend to secrete larger, more buoyant TG-enriched VLDL, and studies suggest that because of a higher TG content, these VLDL are more likely to become TG-enriched LDL, which will then generate small, dense LDL [53].

Many, but not all, cohort studies and post-hoc analyses of clinical trials suggest that small, dense LDL may be particularly atherogenic. However, all of the apoB-lipoproteins, except nascent chylomicrons, have been demonstrated to enter the subendothelial space and accumulate in atherosclerotic lesions. On the other hand, for any plasma LDL cholesterol concentration, a patient with small, dense LDL has more LDL particles, and it is the number of apoB-lipoproteins that is critical in terms of atherogenic risk.

Diabetic dyslipidemia: high-density lipoprotein metabolism and function

HDL is perhaps the most heterogeneous lipoprotein class. Much of this heterogeneity derives from the participation of HDL in RCT [54]. This process initially involves the precursor forms pre-α and pre-β HDL, which very likely represent newly secreted phospholipid discs with apoA-I on the surface. The ATP cassette binding protein A1 (ABCA1) is a cellular transport protein that plays a critical role in transferring intracellular or plasma membrane cholesterol to these nascent, lipid-poor forms of HDL [55]. Transfer (possibly cosecretory) of cholesterol from hepatocytes and intestinal mucosal cells to newly secreted apoA-I/phospholipid discs stabilizes the apoA-I and prolongs its lifespan in the circulation, allowing repetitive cycles of ABCA1-mediated cholesterol efflux to occur, probably from the liver, intestine, and tissues throughout the body, including macrophages containing cholesteryl esters derived from apoB-lipoproteins. Repeated transfer of cholesterol to the surface of the apoA-I/phospholipid disc is coupled with cholesterol esterification by the enzyme lecithin cholesterol acyltransferase (LCAT), allowing the newly generated cholesteryl esters to move from the surface to the core of what then becomes a spherical HDL_3. ApoA-I plays another important role in the formation of HDL_3 through its activation of LCAT. Further accumulation of cholesteryl esters in the core of HDL_3 leads to the generation of HDL_2, which in turn can take on additional cholesterol through interactions with the scavenger receptor B-1 (SRB-1) and a second ATP cassette binding protein, ABCG1 [56]. The mature cholesteryl ester–rich HDL_2 particles are capable of delivering their free and esterified cholesterol to the liver through additional interactions with SRB-1. Of critical importance to RCT is the ability of HDL_2 to deliver free and esterified cholesterol to hepatocytes, without degradation of apoA-I. In fact, evidence indicates that apoA-I can return to the circulation after interacting with SRB-1 as a nascent HDL that can take part in another cycle of RCT.

Alternatively, HDL_2 particles can participate in the CETP-mediated exchange of their cholesteryl esters for TG in chylomicrons, VLDL, and their remnants [57]. The impact of this exchange on RCT is unclear. Removing from the liver the TG-rich lipoproteins that receive the cholesteryl esters from HDL may have no effect on RCT, assuming that delivery of cholesteryl ester by way of uptake of apoB-lipoproteins results in delivery of the lipid to the biliary tract with the same efficiency as does delivery by way of SRB-1. Unfortunately, increased CETP-mediated exchange of HDL cholesteryl esters for TG is associated with lipolysis of HDL TG by HL, and this produces a small, lipid-depleted HDL that resembles the nascent particle. ApoA-I binding to this HDL particle is diminished, causing apoA-I to dissociate from the particle and be cleared more rapidly from the plasma, reducing the number of HDL particles in the circulation. Additionally, if the cholesteryl ester–enriched apoB-lipoproteins are not removed by the liver, but rather, find their way into the artery wall, then the RCT will have been "short circuited" by a futile cycle, and atherogenesis may be accelerated.

HDL cholesterol and apoA-I levels are characteristically reduced in insulin-resistant people with or without type 2 diabetes. Much of this derives from the actions of CETP. Increased HL activity in insulin resistance, with increased hydrolysis of TG and the generation of smaller HDL, may also play a role in this scheme. Thus, fractional catabolism of apoA-I is increased in patients who have type 2 diabetes mellitus [58]. Although apoA-I levels are reduced consistently, correction of hypertriglyceridemia does not usually normalize them, suggesting that other mechanisms are at play. Whether defective ABCA-1–mediated efflux of cellular-free cholesterol, defective LCAT activity, or increased selective delivery of HDL cholesteryl ester to hepatocytes is involved in the low HDL levels present in insulin resistance is under investigation. However, the observation that low HDL cholesterol and apoA-I are present frequently, even when TG levels are relatively normal suggests that non-CETP mechanisms are also important in the pathogenesis of low HDL cholesterol concentrations.

Diabetic dyslipidemia: reducing risk of cardiovascular disease

The importance of diabetes as a risk factor for cardiovascular disease is reflected in its designation as a CHD risk equivalent by the National Cholesterol Education Program Expert Panel in its Adult Treatment Panel (ATP III) report [59,60]. The recommendations of the American Diabetes Association are similar. The cornerstone of evidence-based primary and secondary prevention of CHD is reduction of LDL cholesterol levels to less than 100 mg/dl. This goal should be achieved through therapeutic lifestyle changes (TLC), accompanied by drug therapy if necessary. If LDL cholesterol is greater than or equal to 130 mg/dl at baseline, TLC should be initiated along with drug therapy. For LDL levels between 100 and 129 mg/dl at baseline, TLC remains vital, but clinical judgment may dictate drug treatment. If LDL levels are less than 100 mg/dl at baseline, there are no clear indications for drug therapy for primary prevention. However, a recent white paper from ATP III suggested that patients who have type 2 diabetes who had a prior cardiovascular event were at very high risk; the optimal LDL for that group, according to this new statement, might be less than 70 mg/dl. Therapy with HMG CoA reductase inhibitors (statins) was recommended for this group. ATP III has not set goals for TG and HDL cholesterol levels, whereas the ADA has suggested targets of less than 150 mg/dl for TG and more than 40 mg/dl for HDL (more than 50 mg/dl for women).

A detailed review of dietary and drug therapies for diabetic dyslipidemia is beyond the scope of this article. However, it is clear that weight loss and exercise must play central roles in both short-term and long-term treatment programs. The composition of the diet is not as important during the initial phases of treatment as the caloric intake, although limits on both simple and low-fiber complex carbohydrates are logical in terms of glycemic control. Reductions in saturated and transfatty acids will lower LDL cholesterol 5% to 15%, depending on the individual and the pretreatment diet; replacement of those FA with either monounsaturated or polyunsaturated FA will be equally efficacious. LDL cholesterol can be reduced dramatically by statin therapy, and most of the available statins have demonstrated efficacy for reducing cardiovascular disease in patients who have diabetes (Table 3). Whether the LDL cholesterol goal is less than 100 mg/dl or less than 70 mg/dl, physicians should strive to achieve a reduction of at least 35% to 40% in the concentration of LDL cholesterol; the recent Treat to New Targets study [61] indicates that greater reductions are associated with lower event rates. Nonstatin approaches include bile acid binding resins, which can lower LDL cholesterol by 15% to 20%; stanol or sterol esters from plants (1–3 g per day), which can lower LDL cholesterol by 10% to 15%; and inhibitors of cholesterol absorption from the intestine. This last category has only one available agent, ezetimibe, which reduces LDL cholesterol by 15% to 20%. All these agents appear to be as effective in patients who have diabetes as in the rest of the population.

When dietary change and weight loss are inadequate to reach target levels of HDL cholesterol and TG, treatment has typically meant the use of fibrates and niacin. Gemfibrozil and fenofibrate are the two available fibrates in the United States. These agents are agonists of the peroxisomal proliferator-activated receptor alpha (PPARα) and act mainly to increase FA oxidation in the liver and increase the expression of LpL and apoA-I. Thus, fibrates decrease VLDL TG secretion, improve VLDL and chylomicron TG clearance, and raise HDL cholesterol by reducing TG levels and increasing apoA-I synthesis. In the Veterans Administration HDL Intervention Trial, gemfibrozil was efficacious in reducing cardiovascular events in both nondiabetics and diabetics with prior CHD [62]. In the very recent FIELD trial, fenofibrate was compared with placebo in nearly 10,000 subjects with type 2 diabetes for prevention of cardiovascular events over 5 years: 20% of the participants had had a prior event [63]. Although fenofibrate therapy did not benefit the overall group, there was a 20% reduction in events in participants who had not had a prior event. However, there was no benefit of fenofibrate, compared with placebo, in the group that had had a prior event. A confounding issue in this study was that nearly 40% of the participants on placebo began statin treatment at some point in the study (mean exposure for the group was about 18%), compared with less than 20% of the fenofibrate-treated subjects (mean exposure about 7%). Preliminary evaluation of safety suggested that the combination of statin with fenofibrate (in those whose own physician added a statin during the trial) was safe; myositis did not increase. The ACCORD trial should provide definitive data regarding the efficacy of fenofibrate in this population. In ACCORD, 5500 subjects with diabetes (one half with a prior cardiovascular event) have been randomized to fenofibrate or placebo in the setting of simvastatin therapy (20 or 40 mg/day). The ACCORD trial will be reported in 2009.

Niacin in high doses, between 1000 and 3000 mg/day, can lower LDL cholesterol and TG levels and raise HDL cholesterol concentration. The increases in HDL cholesterol are greater than with any other available agent. In addition, niacin is the most effective agent available for the treatment of high levels of lipoprotein (a). In the Coronary Drug Project, niacin reduced

Table 3
Clinical trials of statin therapy in patients with diabetes mellitus

Trial	NDM (overall)	Treatment (mg/day)	Mean follow-up	% change from baseline			Major CHD[a] Event Rates (%)		RRR % (P value)	ARR (%)	NNT
				LDL cholesterol	TG	HDL cholesterol	Treatment	Placebo			
Secondary prevention											
4S [69]	202 (4444)	Simvastatin 20–40	5.4 y (median)	−36%	−11%	+7%	22.9	45.4	55 (.002)	22.5	4
4S [70]	483 (4398)	Simvastatin 20–40	5.4 y (median)	~ −36%	~ −11%	~ +6%	23.5	37.5	42 (.001)	14.0	7
CARE [71]	586 (4159)	Pravastatin 40	5.0 y	−27	−13	+4	17.7[b]	20.4[b]	13 (NS)	2.7	37
							28.7	36.8	25 (.05)	8.1	12
LIPID [72]	NDM: 1077 IFG: 940	Pravastatin 40	6.0 y	~ −28	~ −19	~ +4	19.6	23.4	DM: 19 (.11)	3.8	26
							11.8	17.8	IFG: 36 (.009)	6.0	17
HPS [73]	5963 (20536)	Simvastatin 40	4.8 y	−28	−13	+1	9.4[c]	12.6[c]	27 (<.0001)	3.2	31
							20.2	25.1	22 (<.0001)	4.9	20
Primary prevention											
ASCOT-LLA [74]	2532 (10305)	Atorvastatin 10	3.3 y (median)	−33[d]	−22[d]	0[d]	3.0	3.6	16 (.43)	0.6	167
CARDS [75]	2838 (2838)	Atorvastatin 10	3.9 y (median)	−31	−17	−9	5.8[e]	9.0[e]	37% (.001)	3.2	31

Abbreviations: ARR, absolute risk reduction; CHD, coronary heart disease; IFG, impaired fasting glucose; NDM, number of patients with diabetes mellitus; NNT, number needed to treat to prevent 1 event; NS, not significant; RRR, relative risk reduction.

[a] Combined coronary death and nonfatal MI unless otherwise specifically noted (see below).

[b] Combined major CHD events, coronary artery bypass graft, percutaneous transluminal coronary angioplasty.

[c] Combined major CHD events, stroke, revascularization.

[d] For overall population.

[e] Combined major CHD events unstable angina, nonfatal cardiac arrest.

recurrent fatal and nonfatal myocardial infarctions during the study, and was associated with greater survival 8 years later [76]. The use of niacin in patients who have type 2 diabetes has been limited by demonstrated increases in insulin resistance and plasma glucose levels during therapy. However, recent studies indicate that when diabetes is well-controlled, the negative effects of niacin on glycemic control can be offset by titration of the diabetes medications already in use [64]. Niacin can, therefore, be considered for patients who have type 2 diabetes and very low levels of HDL cholesterol, although not as a first-line agent. However, the patient must first have good glycemic control and the physician must be willing to monitor the patient carefully and change the diabetes regimen if needed.

Finally, thiazolidinediones (TZDs), which are PPARγ agonists, have, in addition to their glucose-lowering effects, beneficial effects on plasma lipids. Although pioglitazone and rosiglitazone, the two TZDs available in the United States, increase HDL cholesterol and the size and buoyancy of LDL particles, they differ in their effects on TG; only pioglitazone reduces TG levels [65]. In a recent study, the authors demonstrated that the TG lowering with pioglitazone was caused by increased VLDL TG lipolysis secondary to increased LpL and decreased production of apoC-III. The basis for the lack of TG lowering with rosiglitazone is unclear. In the recently published PROACTIVE study [66], pioglitazone was compared with placebo, on the background of standard care, in approximately 5000 subjects with diabetes who had already suffered at least one prior cardiovascular event. There was a 10% reduction (not statistically significant) in a large composite of cardiovascular end points. When the authors examined a smaller cluster of major end points, consisting of all cause mortality, nonfatal myocardial infarction, and stroke, pioglitazone treatment was associated with a 16% reduction of events, compared with placebo ($P = .027$). Hospitalizations for congestive heart failure in the pioglitazone group were 50% higher than in the placebo group (absolute rates: 6% versus 4%). However, the pioglitazone group showed no increase in mortality from congestive heart failure. Further studies of the efficacy of PPARγ agonists for the prevention of cardiovascular disease are needed.

Summary

Diabetes mellitus, particularly type 2 diabetes, is associated with a markedly increased risk of cardiovascular disease. Much of this increased risk derives from a complex dyslipidemia that is an integral part of the underlying insulin resistance present in this group, and which can be exacerbated by insulin deficiency. Overproduction of VLDL is a central feature of the diabetic dyslipidemia, and this accounts for much of the low HDL and abnormal LDL also present. A number of physiologic and pharmacologic approaches are available and should be used aggressively to treat the diabetic dyslipidemia.

References

[1] Centers for Disease Control and Prevention. National diabetes fact sheet: general information and national estimates on diabetes in the United States, 2005. Atlanta (GA): US Department of Health and Human Services. Centers for Disease Control and Prevention; 2005.

[2] Grundy SM, Benjamin IJ, Burke GL, et al. Diabetes and cardiovascular disease. A statement for healthcare professionals from the American Heart Association. Circulation 1999;100: 1134–46.

[3] Morrish NJ, Wang S-L, Stevens LK. et al, and the WHO Multinational Study Group. Mortality and causes of death in the WHO multinational study of vascular disease in diabetes. Diabetologia 2001;44(Suppl 2):S14–21.

[4] Stamler J, Vaccaro O, Neaton JD, et al. Diabetes, other risk factors, and 12-yr cardiovascular mortality for men screened in the multiple risk factor intervention trial. Diabetes Care 1993;16(2):434–44.

[5] Beckman JA, Creager MA, Libby P. Diabetes and atherosclerosis: epidemiology, pathophysiology, and management. JAMA 2002;287(19):2570–81.

[6] Whiteley L, Padmanabhan S, Hole D, et al. Should diabetes be considered a coronary heart disease risk equivalent? Results from 25 years of follow-up in the Renfrew and Paisley survey. Diabetes Care 2005;28(7):1588–93.

[7] Haffner SM, Lehto S, Rönnemaa T, et al. Mortality from coronary heart disease in subjects with type 2 diabetes and in nondiabetic subjects with and without prior myocardial infarction. N Engl J Med 1998;339(4):229–34.

[8] Becker A, Bos G, de Vegt F, et al. Cardiovascular events in type 2 diabetes: comparison with nondiabetic individuals without and with prior cardiovascular disease. 10-year follow-up of the Hoorn study. Eur Heart J 2003;24:1406–13.

[9] Miettinen H, Lehto S, Salomaa V, et al. Impact of diabetes on mortality after the first myocardial infarction. The FINMONICA myocardial infarction register study group. Diabetes Care 1998;21(1):69–75.

[10] Howard BV, Rodriguez BL, Bennett PH, et al. Prevention conference VI. Diabetes and cardiovascular disease writing group I: epidemiology. Circulation 2002;105:e132–7.

[11] Mak K-H, Haffner SM. Diabetes abolishes the gender gap in coronary heart disease. Eur Heart J 2003;24:1385–6.

[12] Howard BV, Cowan LD, Go O, et al, for the Strong Heart Study investigators. Adverse effects of diabetes on multiple cardiovascular disease risk factors in women. The Strong Heart Study. Diabetes Care 1998;21(8):1258–65.

[13] Juutilainen A, Kortelainen S, Lehto S, et al. Gender difference in the impact of type 2 diabetes on coronary heart disease risk. Diabetes Care 2004;27(12):2898–904.

[14] Ginsberg HN. Lipoprotein physiology in nondiabetic and diabetic states: relationship to atherogenesis. Diabetes Care 1991;14:839–55.

[15] Kreisberg RA. Diabetic dyslipidemia. Am J Cardiol 1998;82:67U–73U.

[16] Haffner SM. Lipoprotein disorders associated with type 2 diabetes mellitus and insulin resistance. Am J Cardiol 2002;90(suppl):55i–61i.

[17] Ebara T, Conde K, Kako Y, et al. Delayed catabolism of apoB-48 lipoproteins due to decreased heparan sulfate proteoglycan production in diabetic mice. J Clin Invest 2000; 105(12):1807–18.

[18] Brunzell JD. Increased ApoB in small dense LDL particles predicts premature coronary artery disease. Arterioscler Thromb Vasc Biol 2005;25(3):474–5.

[19] Krauss RM. Lipids and lipoproteins in patients with type 2 diabetes. Diabetes Care 2004; 27(6):1496–504.

[20] Sacks FM, Campos H. Clinical review 163: Cardiovascular endocrinology: low-density lipoprotein size and cardiovascular disease: a reappraisal. J Clin Endocrinol Metab 2003;88(10): 4525–32.

[21] Haidari M, Leung N, Mahbub F, et al. Fasting and postprandial overproduction of intestinally derived lipoproteins in an animal model of insulin resistance. Evidence that chronic fructose feeding in the hamster is accompanied by enhanced intestinal de novo lipogenesis and ApoB48-containing lipoprotein overproduction. J Biol Chem 2002;277:31646–55.

[22] Pennacchio LA, Rubin EM. Apolipoprotein A5, a newly identified gene that affects plasma triglyceride levels in humans and mice. Arterioscler Thromb Vasc Biol 2003;23(4):529–34 [Epub 2002 Dec].

[23] Cianflone K, Xia Z, Chen LY. Critical review of acylation-stimulating protein physiology in humans and rodents. Biochim Biophys Acta 2003;1609(2):127–43.

[24] Merkel M, Eckel RH, Goldberg IJ. Lipoprotein lipase: genetics, lipid uptake, and regulation. J Lipid Res 2002;43:1997–2006.

[25] Altomonte J, Cong L, Harbaran S, et al. Foxo1 mediates insulin action on apoC-III and triglyceride metabolism. J Clin Invest 2004;114:1493–503.

[26] Cohn JS, Patterson BW, Uffelman KD, et al. Rate of production of plasma and very-low-density lipoprotein (VLDL) apolipoprotein C–III is strongly related to the concentration and level of production of VLDL triglyceride in male subjects with different body weights and levels of insulin sensitivity. J Clin Endocrinol Metab 2004;89:3949–55.

[27] Nowak M, Helleboid-Chapman A, Jakel H, et al. Insulin-mediated down-regulation of apolipoprotein A5 gene expression through the phosphatidylinositol 3-kinase pathway: role of upstream stimulatory factor. Mol Cell Biol 2005;25(4):1537–48.

[28] Brunzell JD, Hazzard WR, Porte D Jr, et al. Evidence for a common, saturable, triglyceride removal mechanism for chylomicrons and very low density lipoproteins in man. J Clin Invest 1973;52(7):1578–85.

[29] Bjorkegren J, Packard CJ, Hamsten A, et al. Accumulation of large very low density lipoprotein in plasma during intravenous infusion of a chylomicron-like triglyceride emulsion reflects competition for a common lipolytic pathway. J Lipid Res 1996;37:76–86.

[30] Shachter N. Apolipoproteins C–I and C–III as important modulators of lipoprotein metabolism. Curr Opin Lipidol 2001;12(3):297–304.

[31] Kissebah AH. Low density lipoprotein metabolism in non-insulin-dependent diabetes mellitus. Diabetes Metab Rev 1987;3:619–51.

[32] Zambon A, Bertocco S, Vitturi N, et al. Relevance of hepatic lipase to the metabolism of triacylglycerol-rich lipoproteins. Biochem Soc Trans 2003;31:1070–4.

[33] Ginsberg HN, Illingworth DR. Postprandial dyslipidemia: an atherogenic disorder common in patients with diabetes mellitus. Am J Cardiol 2001;88(suppl):9H–15H.

[34] Olofsson SO, Stillemark-Billton P, Asp L. Intracellular assembly of VLDL: two major steps in separate cell compartments. Trends Cardiovasc Med 2000;10:338–45.

[35] Fisher EA, Ginsberg HN. Complexity in the secretory pathway: the assembly and secretion of apolipoprotein B-containing lipoproteins. J Biol Chem 2002;277:17377–80.

[36] Fisher EA, Pan M, Chen X, et al. The triple threat to nascent apolipoprotein B. Evidence for multiple, distinct degradative pathways. J Biol Chem 2001;276(30):27855–63.

[37] Ginsberg HN. Insulin resistance and cardiovascular disease. J Clin Invest 2000;106:453–8.

[38] Kissebah AH, Alfarsi S, Adams PW, et al. Role of insulin resistance in adipose tissue and liver in the pathogenesis of endogenous hypertriglyceridaemia in man. Diabetologia 1976; 12:563–71.

[39] Lewis GF. Fatty acid regulation of very low density lipoprotein (VLDL) production. Curr Opin Lipidol 1999;10:475–7.

[40] Zhang Y, Ono-Hernandez A, Ko C, et al. Regulation of hepatic lipoprotein assembly and secretion by the availability of fatty acids. I: Differential responses to the delivery of fatty acids via albumin or remnant-like emulsion particles. J Biol Chem 2004;279: 19362–74.

[41] Craig WY, Nutik R, Cooper AD. Regulation of apoprotein synthesis and secretion in the human hepatoma Hep G2. The effect of exogenous lipoprotein. J Biol Chem 1988;263: 13880–90.

[42] Cohn JS, Wagner DA, Cohn SD, et al. Measurement of very low density and low density li-
     poprotein apolipoprotein (Apo) B-100 and high density lipoprotein Apo A-I production in
     human subjects using deuterated leucine. Effect of fasting and feeding. J Clin Invest 1990;85:
     804–11.
[43] Schwarz JM, Linfoot P, Dare D, et al. Hepatic de novo lipogenesis in normoinsulinemic and
     hyperinsulinemic subjects consuming high-fat, low-carbohydrate and low-fat, high-carbohy-
     drate isoenergetic diets. Am J Clin Nutr 2003;77:43–50.
[44] Donnelly KL, Smith CI, Schwarzenberg SJ, et al. Sources of fatty acids stored in liver and
     secreted via lipoproteins in patients with nonalcoholic fatty liver disease. J Clin Invest
     2005;115(5):1343–51.
[45] Horton JD, Goldstein JL, Brown MS. SREBPs: activators of the complete program of
     cholesterol and fatty acidsynthesis in the liver. J Clin Invest 2002;109:1125–31.
[46] Shimomura I, Matsuda M, Hammer RE, et al. Decreased IRS-2 and increased SREBP-1c
     lead to mixed insulin resistance and sensitivity in livers of lipodystrophic and ob/ob mice.
     Mol Cell 2000;6:77–86.
[47] Siri P, Candela N, Ko C, et al. Post-transcriptional stimulation of the assembly and secretion
     of triglyceride-rich apolipoproteinB-lipoproteins in a mouse with selective deficiency of
     brown adipose tissue, obesity and insulin resistance. J Biol Chem 2001;276:46064–72.
[48] Sparks JD, Sparks CE. Insulin regulation of triacylglycerol-rich lipoprotein synthesis and
     secretion. Biochim Biophys Acta 1994;1215(1–2):9–32.
[49] Pan M, Cederbaum AI, Zhang Y-L, et al. Lipid peroxidation and oxidant stress regulate he-
     patic apolipoprotein B degradation and VLDL production. J Clin Invest 2004;113:1277–88.
[50] Lewis GF, Uffelman KD, Szeto LW, et al. Effects of acute hyperinsulinemia on VLDL tri-
     glyceride and VLDL apoB production in normal weight and obese individuals. Diabetes
     1993;42:833–42.
[51] Malmstrom R, Packard CJ, Caslake M, et al. Defective regulation of triglyceride metabolism
     by insulin in the liver in NIDDM. Diabetologia 1997;40:454–62.
[52] Austin MA, Krauss RM. LDL density and atherosclerosis. JAMA 1995;273:115.
[53] Krauss RM, Siri PW. Metabolic abnormalities: triglyceride and low-density lipoprotein. En-
     docrinol Metab Clin North Am 2004;33(2):405–15.
[54] Lewis GF, Rader DJ. New insights into the regulation of HDL metabolism and reverse cho-
     lesterol transport. Circ Res 2005;96(12):1221–32.
[55] Oram JF, Heinecke JW. ATP-binding cassette transporter A1: a cell cholesterol exporter
     that protects against cardiovascular disease. Physiol Rev 2005;85(4):1343–72.
[56] Wang N, Lan D, Chen W, et al. ATP-binding cassette transporters G1 and G4 mediate cel-
     lular cholesterol efflux to high-density lipoproteins. Proc Natl Acad Sci USA 2004;101(26):
     9774–9.
[57] Stein O, Stein Y. Lipid transfer proteins (LTP) and atherosclerosis. Atherosclerosis 2005;
     178(2):217–30.
[58] Horowitz BS, Goldberg IJ, Merab J, et al. Increased plasma and renal clearance of an ex-
     changeable pool of apolipoprotein A-I in subjects with low levels of high density lipoprotein
     cholesterol. J Clin Invest 1993;91:1743–60.
[59] Cleeman JI, Expert Panel on Detection, Evaluation, and Treatment of High Blood Cho-
     lesterol In Adults. Executive summary of the third report of the National Cholesterol
     Education Program (NCEP) Expert Panel on Detection, Evaluation, and Treatment of
     High Blood Cholesterol in Adults (Adult Treatment Panel III). JAMA 2001;285(19):
     2486–97.
[60] Third report of the National Cholesterol Education Program (NCEP) Expert Panel on
     Detection. Evaluation, and Treatment of High Blood Cholesterol in Adults (Adult Treat-
     ment Panel III). Final report. NIH Publication No. 02–5215. Circulation 2002;106(25):
     3143–421.
[61] LaRosa JC, Grundy SM, Waters DD. Intensive lipid lowering with atorvastatin in patients
     with stable coronary disease. N Engl J Med 2005;352:1425–35.

[62] Rubins HB, Robbins SJ, Collins P, et al, for the Veterans Affairs High-Density Lipoprotein Cholesterol Intervention Trial Study group. Gemfibrozil for the secondary prevention of coronary heart disease in men with low levels of high-density lipoprotein cholesterol. N Engl J Med 1999;341:410–8.

[63] Keech A, Simes RJ, Barter P, et al, for the FIELD study investigators. Effects of long-term fenofibrate therapy on cardiovascular events in 9795 people with type 2 diabetes mellitus (the FIELD study): randomised controlled trial. Lancet 2005;366(9500):1849–61.

[64] Meyers CD, Kashyap ML. Management of the metabolic syndrome-nicotinic acid. Endocrinol Metab Clin North Am 2004;33:557–75.

[65] Goldberg RB, Kendall DM, Deeg MA, et al, for the GLAI Study Investigators. A comparison of lipid and glycemic effects of pioglitazone and rosiglitazone in patients with type 2 diabetes and dyslipidemia. Diabetes Care 2005;28(7):1547–54.

[66] Dormandy JA, Charbonnel B, Eckland DJ, et al, for the PROactive investigators. Secondary prevention of macrovascular events in patients with type 2 diabetes in the PROactive Study (PROspective pioglitAzone Clinical Trial In macroVascular Events): a randomised controlled trial. Lancet 2005;366(9493):1279–89.

[67] Wei M, Gaskill SP, Haffner SM, et al. Effects of diabetes and level of glycemia on all-cause and cardiovascular mortality. The San Antonio Heart Study. Diabetes Care 1998;21(7): 1167–72.

[68] Siegel RD, Cupples A, Schaefer EJ, et al. Lipoproteins, apolipoproteins, and low-density lipoprotein size among diabetics in the Framingham Offspring Study. Metabolism 1996; 45(10):1267–72.

[69] Pyörälä K, Pedersen TR, Kjekshus J, et al. Cholesterol lowering with simvastatin improves prognosis of diabetic patients with coronary heart disease: a subgroup analysis of the Scandinavian Simvastatin Survival Study (4S). Diabetes Care 1997;20:614–20.

[70] Haffner SM, Alexander CM, Cook TJ, et al. Reduced coronary events in simvastatin-treated patients with coronary heart disease and diabetes or impaired fasting glucose levels: subgroup analyses in the Scandinavian Simvastatin Survival Study. Arch Intern Med 1999; 159:2661–7.

[71] Goldberg RB, Mellies MJ, Sacks FM, et al. Cardiovascular events and their reduction with pravastatin in diabetic and glucose-intolerant myocardial infarction survivors with average cholesterol levels: subgroup analyses in the Cholesterol and Recurrent Events (CARE) trial. Circulation 1998;98:2513–9.

[72] Keech A, Colquhoun D, Best J, et al, for the LIPID Study Group. Secondary prevention of cardiovascular events with long-term pravastatin in patients with diabetes or impaired fasting glucose: results from the LIPID trial. Diabetes Care 2003;26:2713–21.

[73] Heart Protection Study Collaborative Group. MRC/BHF Heart Protection Study of cholesterol-lowering with simvastatin in 5963 people with diabetes: a randomised placebo-controlled trial. Lancet 2003;361:2005–16.

[74] Sever PS, Dahlöf B, Poulter NR, et al, for the ASCOT investigators. Prevention of coronary and stroke events with atorvastatin in hypertensive patients who have average or lower-than-average cholesterol concentrations, in the Anglo-Scandinavian Cardiac Outcomes Trial - Lipid Lowering Arm (ASCOT-LLA): a multicentre randomised controlled trial. Lancet 2003;361:1149–57.

[75] Colhoun HM, Betteridge DJ, Durrington PN, et al. for the CARDS investigators. Primary prevention of cardiovascular disease with atorvastatin in type 2 diabetes in the Collaborative Atorvastatin Diabetes Study (CARDS): multicentre randomised placebo-controlled trial. Lancet 2004;364:685–96.

[76] Canner PL, Berge KG, Wenger NK, et al. Fifteen year mortality in coronary drug project patients: long-term benefit with niacin. J Am Coll Cardiol 1986;8:1245–55.

ELSEVIER
SAUNDERS

Endocrinol Metab Clin N Am
35 (2006) 511–524

ENDOCRINOLOGY
AND METABOLISM
CLINICS
OF NORTH AMERICA

Receptor for Advanced Glycation End Products and the Cardiovascular Complications of Diabetes and Beyond: Lessons from AGEing

Shi Fang Yan, MD, Shi Du Yan, MD,
Kevan Herold, MD, Ravichandran Ramsamy, PhD,
Ann Marie Schmidt, MD*

*Columbia University Medical Center, 630 West 168th Street, P&S 17-501,
New York, NY 10032, USA*

The presence of elevated blood glucose levels characterizes the diabetic state. Although hyperglycemia may be caused by a number of underlying factors, from frank insulin deficiency consequent to autoimmune destruction of the islets of the pancreas, to severe insulin resistance, the consequences of chronically elevated glucose are remarkably similar. Both the macrovasculature and the microvasculature are exquisitely sensitive to the long-term effects of elevated blood glucose. Among the numerous complications of diabetes, cardiovascular disease remains the leading cause of morbidity and mortality, regardless of the underlying cause of hyperglycemia [1–4]. This article focuses on the impact of Advanced Glycation End products (AGEs), the products of nonenzymatic glycation and the oxidation that occurs consequent to the effects of glucose on the modification of vulnerable lysine or arginine groups of proteins. Although other substrates, such as DNA, are also susceptible to glycation, this article addresses the impact of nonenzymatic glycation on the proteome. The impact of AGEs on the alteration of protein function and signal transduction mechanisms contributes to complications in diabetes. This suggests that blocking the generation or molecular impact of AGEs may modulate the complications of diabetes, in both the macro- and microvasculature.

* Corresponding author.
E-mail address: ams11@columbia.edu (A.M. Schmidt).

0889-8529/06/$ - see front matter © 2006 Elsevier Inc. All rights reserved.
doi:10.1016/j.ecl.2006.06.003

Advanced glycation end products (sparks in the pathogenesis of diabetic complications): generation and interaction with receptor for age

Evidence suggests that AGE formation and accumulation are increased in diabetes [5]. Glycation adducts of proteins form when proteins react with glucose-reactive alpha oxoaldehydes, such as glyoxal, methylglyoxal, and 3-deoxyglucosone [6]. Initial Schiff base adducts, formed from glucose, lysine, and N-terminal amino acid residues, may rearrange to form intermediates, which after further rearrangements, may form AGEs.

In addition to being caused by hyperglycemia, AGEs may be formed directly by inflammatory mechanisms. For example, studies have demonstrated that activating the myeloperoxidase pathway directly generates the specific AGE, carboxymethyl (lysine) (CML-AGE) [7]. In addition, increased oxidative stress is a key characteristic in such settings as hyperglycemia, inflammation, aging, and renal failure, and has been linked to AGE generation [8]. It is conceivable that in stress conditions, AGEs beget oxidative stress, thereby providing a mechanism not only for tissue injury, but for further generation of AGEs.

AGEs may be either fluorescent or nonfluorescent and may cross-link proteins, thereby altering properties that affect permeability and cellular motility. A diverse array of AGE products has been detected and characterized in vivo, such as bis(lysyl)imidazolium cross-links, hydroimidazolones, and monolysyl adducts. Other AGEs that are highly prevalent in diabetes, such as CML-AGEs, may form [9–12].

In addition to the effects of AGE-mediated cross-linking or proteins, AGEs may activate signal transduction mechanisms, thereby changing the properties of cultured cells or animal model systems. The chief cell surface receptor for AGEs is the receptor for advanced glycation end products (RAGE), a member of the immunoglobulin superfamily [13,14]. RAGE has been expressed on a range of cell types implicated in diabetic complications, and in cultured systems the interaction of AGEs with RAGE modulated certain cellular properties. In endothelial cells, AGE–RAGE interaction modulated expression of adhesion molecules and of proinflammatory molecules such as Vascular Cell Adhesion Molecule-1 (VCAM); in fibroblasts, AGE–RAGE interaction affected collagen production; in smooth muscle cells (SMC), AGE–RAGE interaction modulated migration, proliferation, and expression of matrix-modifying molecules; in mononuclear phagocytes, AGE–RAGE interaction stimulated chemotaxis, haptotaxis and expression of proinflammatory molecules; and in lymphocytes, AGE–RAGE interaction enhanced proliferation and generation of IL-2 [15–19].

A chief way, at least in part, in which AGE–RAGE interaction modulates cellular properties is through the generation of oxidative stress. Experimental evidence suggests that reactive oxygen species (ROS), generated through the interaction of RAGE with AGEs, occurs through both activation of NADPH oxidase and recruitment of the mitochondrial electron transport systems that produce these species [20–23].

In the first studies, in vitro–prepared AGEs were used to identify and probe the impact of the interaction of AGEs with RAGE. AGEs on the surface of diabetic red blood cells (RBCs) were used to address the issue of the relevance of these prepared AGEs to the in vivo setting. Cultured ECs bound diabetic RBCs in a manner blocked by excess AGE-bovine serum albumin, anti-AGE immunoglobulin G (IgG), or anti-RAGE IgG. Diabetic RBC AGEs, by way of RAGE, enhanced the generation of ROS and upregulated the expression of VCAM-1 [24,25]. Further, efforts to identify specific AGEs that bound and activated RAGE led to the observation that CML-AGEs interacted with this receptor. In radioligand binding assays, CML-modified AGEs bound RAGE in a dose-dependent and saturable manner. Further, CML-ovalbumin, incubated with cultured endothelial cells, upregulated expression of VCAM-1 and activated NF-kB [26]. These effects were blocked by the addition of neutralizing antibodies to RAGE or the introduction of signal transduction deficient mutants of RAGE, dominant negative RAGE [26].

Taken together, these studies indicated that AGEs bound RAGE and modulated the properties of key cells implicated in the pathogenesis of diabetes-associated complications.

Receptor for advanced glycation end products is a multi-ligand receptor: implications for inflammatory mechanisms in diabetes complications

S100/calgranulins

Studies have demonstrated that RAGE, in addition to AGEs, interacts with distinct ligands. Among these are the proinflammatory S100/calgranulins, which are composed of a family of at least 20 different polypeptides. The principal function of these molecules involves intracellular calcium binding. S100/calgranulins may be expressed in a wide array of cell types, such as polymorphonuclear leukocytes, dendritic cells, mononuclear phagocyte, and lymphocytes [27]. The authors' studies have shown that at least some of the S100/calgranulin family, including S100A12, S100B, and S100P, bind RAGE [28,29]. Although S100/calgranulins are intracellular molecules, studies indicate that these species may be released by cells into the extracellular environment, thereby facilitating their interaction with cell surface RAGE [30,31].

High mobility group box 1 (amphoterin)

High mobility group box 1 (HMGB1), or amphoterin, possesses important functions within the cell as a DNA binding protein. HMGB1 may exist in the extracellular space and on the surface of cells, especially those cells actively involved in migration [32]. Studies have indicated that HMGB1 interacts with RAGE; in early experiments, HGMB1–RAGE interaction was linked to neurite outgrowth and tumor growth and metastases [33,34]. Other studies linked HMGB1 directly to inflammation. Analogous to the biology of S100/calgranulins, HMGB1 may be released from activated cells such as MP, thereby leading to propagation of inflammatory responses [35]. In vivo, administration of blocking antibodies to HMGB1 enhanced the survival of rodents subjected to overwhelming septic shock [35]. These findings suggest important roles for HMGB1 in magnifying proinflammatory mechanisms.

Although it has been shown that HMGB1 may also interact with toll-like receptors 2 and 4, it is clear that the blockade of RAGE attenuates proinflammatory mechanisms in vivo. In euglycemic mice, blockade of RAGE, genetic deletion of RAGE, or transgenic expression of dominant negative RAGE suppressed delayed-type hypersensitivity in mice sensitized and challenged with methylated bovine serum albumin; decreased colonic inflammation in IL-10 deficient mice; suppressed experimental autoimmune encephalomyelitis in mice exposed to encephalitogenic T cells and myelin basic protein; prolonged the time to hyperglycemia in NOD/scid mice treated with diabetogenic splenocytes; increased survival consequent to massive sepsis; and suppressed joint inflammation and destruction in DBA/1 mice sensitized and challenged with bovine type II collagen [28,36–39].

Roles for S100/calgranulins in diabetic inflammatory stress were suggested by the observation that S100/calgranulin expression was high in diabetic macrovessels in a murine model [40]. Experimental evidence from human subjects placed these ligands in the context of diabetes or cardiovascular disease as well. Levels of S100A12 were increased in the plasma of subjects with type 2 diabetes, and increased expression of HMGB1 was observed in human atherosclerotic lesions, particularly in mononuclear phagocytes [41,42].

Other studies indicated that amyloid-beta peptide, beta sheet fibrils, the integrin, Mac-1, bound RAGE [43–45]. Taken together, these findings suggest that RAGE interaction with inflammatory and oxidative stress-provoking ligands might contribute to the pathogenesis of vascular complications in diabetes.

Receptor for advanced glycation end products: at the right place and time in human diabetes and cardiovascular disease

Given the increased incidence of cardiovascular disease in subjects who have either type 1 or 2 diabetes, compared with nondiabetic control subjects, it was logical to assess the levels of RAGE in this disorder. Studies of human carotid artery plaques have suggested that RAGE is expressed in both diabetic and nondiabetic atherosclerotic vessels [46]. However, by both immunohistochemistry and western blotting, it was shown that RAGE was expressed more in the diabetic lesions. RAGE colocalized with inflammatory and oxidative stress markers in these atherosclerotic plaques [46].

Recent studies have now identified that in addition to tissue levels of RAGE, soluble (s) forms of RAGE may be detectable in the plasma of human subjects. In Italian men without diabetes, endogenously lower levels of sRAGE were associated with an enhanced risk of angiographically documented coronary artery disease. Further, individuals with the very lowest levels of sRAGE displayed the greatest overall risk for disease [47]. In another study, it was shown that individuals with essential hypertension displayed significantly lower levels of plasma sRAGE, compared with normotensive subjects [48].

These concepts have been extended to diabetes. Levels of a particular soluble form of RAGE, called endogenous or esRAGE, were decreased in the plasma of subjects with type 1 diabetes and were inversely correlated with the severity of macro- and microvessel perturbation, specifically carotid intima, media thickness, and retinopathy [49]. In one study, sRAGE levels were inversely correlated with components of metabolic syndrome, including body mass index, blood pressure, triglycerides, glycosylated hemoglobin, or insulin resistance index [50]. Modulation of sRAGE levels, coincident with administration of perindopril, was shown by Forbes and colleagues [51]. In these studies, subjects with type 1 diabetes treated with this inhibitor of angiotensin-converting enzyme-1 displayed increased levels of sRAGE after treatment. They identified complexes between sRAGE and CML-adducts in the human diabetic plasma [51].

In the current state of the art, two enzyme-linked immunosorbent assays (ELISAs) are available to measure sRAGE. The identification of the specific splice variant of RAGE (esRAGE) measures a specific variant of the soluble form of the receptor. In another ELISA system, all forms of sRAGE, the extracellular domain of the receptor, are recognized. No direct evidence at this time indicates that in humans, sRAGE may be released based on cleavage of the cell surface receptor. The relationships between total sRAGE and the specific variant esRAGE are not clarified yet.

Studies in human subjects further suggest that genetic variants of RAGE may be associated with risk for coronary artery disease. A particular promoter allele (-374 A) of the gene-encoding RAGE is associated with decreased macrovascular disease in diabetic human subjects [52]. Furthermore, associations of this variant in nondiabetic subjects have been shown as well [53,54]. Although two other reports did not identify modulation of risk for cardiovascular disease in subjects with these variants [55,56], these findings suggested that expression levels of the receptor (driven in this case by promoter variants) may predict, at least in part, vulnerability to coronary artery disease. Thus, larger-scale studies are required to address this question definitively in both the diabetic and nondiabetic state.

In other studies, a distinct variant, RAGE G82S, was studied because the product of this variant lies within the V-type immunoglobulin domain of

RAGE [36]. Thus, it was conceivable that genetic variants in this V-domain might encode proteins that enhance or diminish vulnerability to atherosclerosis. However, analysis of subjects in the Framingham offspring cohort failed to identify specific links of this variant to coronary artery disease, either in diabetes or euglycemia [57].

Taken together, these studies illustrated potential associations of RAGE biology to human diabetes and cardiovascular disease. Yet such studies did not identify if RAGE was more likely a marker of disease or a participant in the pathogenesis of vascular perturbation. To address these concepts, animal models of diabetes and cardiovascular injury were established, and pharmacologic blockade of RAGE or genetic modulation of the receptor were used to test the impact of RAGE.

Animal models of atherosclerosis and restenosis: the impact of the receptor for advanced glycation end products

Atherosclerosis

As a first test of the role of RAGE in vivo in animal models of atherosclerosis, mice deficient in apolipoprotein E were used, because these animals displayed spontaneous hypercholesterolemia and an age-dependent increase in atherosclerotic lesion area and complexity, versus wild-type mice. Induction of relative insulin-deficient (type 1) diabetes in these mice with streptozotocin revealed significantly increased atherosclerosis and vascular inflammation, compared with nondiabetic apoE null mice of the same age [40,58]. To block ligand–RAGE interaction in these animals, a soluble form of RAGE was used. Soluble RAGE was generated and purified in a baculovirus expression system and administered once daily intraperitoneally to apoE null mice rendered diabetic with streptozotocin. Diabetic mice received sRAGE beginning immediately at the time of documentation of hyperglycemia; this was continued for a total of 6 weeks duration. Compared with vehicle (murine serum albumin)–treated mice, sRAGE-treated animals displayed a dose-dependent decrease in atherosclerosis area at the aortic root, and decreased features of lesion complexity [58]. Blockade of RAGE did not affect levels of lipids or glucose, thereby suggesting that RAGE acted downstream of these key risk factors [58].

To test the role of RAGE in diabetic apoE null mice with established atherosclerosis, sRAGE was administered to diabetic mice after 6 weeks of sustained hyperglycemia, and then continued for an additional 6 weeks [59]. Control diabetic animals received murine serum albumin. These studies revealed that sRAGE-treated mice displayed significant stabilization of lesion area and complexity at the aortic root, compared with diabetic mice treated with vehicle [59]. In sRAGE-treated mice, vascular inflammation and oxidant stress were attenuated markedly in the aortae, as reflected by decreased cox-2, nitrotyrosine epitopes, JE-MCP-1, and tissue factor antigens; MMP9 antigen/activity; and phosphorylated p38 MAP kinase [59]. In the animals treated with sRAGE, there were no differences in glucose, insulin, lipid number, or profile [59].

An essential step in these studies was to test the premise that the role of the ligand–RAGE axis in the modulation of diabetic atherosclerosis in murine models was not limited to streptozotocin-induced hyperglycemia. To test the role of RAGE in murine models of type 2 diabetes, apoE null mice were bred into the db/db background. These db/db mice are a model of severe insulin-resistant diabetes based on abnormalities in leptin receptor signaling; in this model, all mice become hyperglycemic by the age of 8 weeks. In apoE null db/db mice, atherosclerosis was accelerated, compared with littermate apoE null mice without diabetes. Further, consistent with key roles for RAGE in atherosclerosis in the diabetic mice, administration of sRAGE from age 8 to 11 weeks resulted in a highly significant decrease in atherosclerotic lesion area, with a decreased vascular expression of S100/calgranulins, VCAM-1, and MMPs [60].

Studies of animal and human models of cardiovascular disease have revealed increased accumulation of RAGE ligands in atherosclerotic plaques, even in the absence of hyperglycemia. Vascular inflammation and oxidative stress clearly may drive generation of AGEs, and may increase expression of proinflammatory S100/calgranulins and HMGB1. Thus, to test the potential role of RAGE in euglycemic atherosclerosis, the authors administered sRAGE to nondiabetic apoE null mice (C57BL/6 background) and to apoE null mice in the db background. In both animal models, sRAGE-treated nondiabetic mice displayed significantly decreased atherosclerosis and vascular inflammation, compared with vehicle-treated control mice [59,60].

These studies confirmed the fundamental premise that although diabetes represents a state of exaggerated ligand generation (even in nondiabetic atherosclerotic disease), oxidative stress, triggered by hyperlipidemia and inflammation, contributes integrally to the pathogenesis of atherosclerosis, at least in part by way of RAGE ligation.

Restenosis

In addition to the exaggerated neointimal expansion characteristic of chronic atherosclerosis, diabetes is associated with increased neointimal expansion consequent to acute vascular injury, such as that triggered by angioplasty. In rodent models, proliferation and migration of SMC are key mediators of an increased intima/media (I/M) ratio consequent to either carotid or femoral artery injury, for example. RAGE is expressed highly in SMC, particularly in those exposed to vascular stress. To date, the role of the RAGE axis in injury-triggered neointimal expansion has been studied in rats and mice.

Specifically, in diabetic Zucker fatty rats, balloon-induced carotid artery injury initiated increased SMC proliferation and significantly increased neointimal thickness 28 days after injury, compared with nondiabetic littermate rats. In these diabetic animals, administration of sRAGE during the first week after injury, corresponding to the peak of SMC proliferation, resulted in significantly decreased intima/media thickness, largely because of decreased SMC proliferation [61].

These concepts were extended to nondiabetes and addressed in C57BL/6 mice. Endothelial denudation was induced by catheters in the femoral artery. Acute injury resulted in a rapid increase in at least two classes of RAGE ligands, AGEs (in particular, CML epitopes) and S100/clagranlulins [17]. Thus, even in the absence of hyperglycemia, physical injury is a potent stimulus that may lead to rapid generation of RAGE ligands, and, in turn, upregulation of RAGE.

Key roles for the ligand–RAGE axis in the pathogenesis of injury-stimulated neointimal expansion have been highlighted using multiple strategies. Administering sRAGE or blocking antibodies to RAGE, compared with respective vehicle treatments, resulted in a significant decrease in I/M ratio. Using genetic approaches, it was shown further that a significantly decreased I/M ratio resulted consequent to femoral artery endothelial denudation in homozygous RAGE null mice or transgenic mice in which signal transduction–deficient mutants of RAGE were expressed selectively in SMC by the SM22 alpha promoter, compared with wild-type littermates [17].

Taken together, these studies indicate that physical injury, either in the diabetic or nondiabetic state, rapidly upregulates RAGE ligands and leads to increased expression and function of RAGE. In the diabetic environment, it is likely that basal upregulation of the ligand–RAGE axis sets the stage for even further exaggeration of SMC proliferation and migration, and, therefore, increased neointimal expansion.

Receptor for advanced glycation end products and inflammation: coming full circle in the pathogenesis of diabetes

The increasing evidence that RAGE was linked to inflammation, even in the absence of diabetes, led to the hypothesis that RAGE was implicated in the pathogenesis of immune damage that results in islet destruction and, therefore, insulin deficiency. The first studies suggesting roles for RAGE in adaptive immunity were performed in a murine model of experimental autoimmune encephalomyelitis in mice exposed to encephalitogenic T cells and myelin basic protein [37]. These concepts were then extended to a murine model of type 1 diabetes in which immune mechanisms linked to pathogenesis might be studied. Thus, the RAGE axis was studied in a model of adoptive transfer of diabetogenic spleen cells into NOD/scid mice. After transfer of these spleen cells, immunohistochemistry revealed that RAGE, and its proinflammatory ligand S100, were expressed on islet cells with an inflammatory infiltrate in sections of pancreata from diabetic NOD/scid mice [38].

To assess pathogenic roles for RAGE, NOD/scid mice received a transfer of splenocytes from a diabetic NOD donor and were treated with either sRAGE or vehicle. Treatment with sRAGE reduced the rate of diabetes transfer significantly and prolonged the time to hyperglycemia. Further, the expression of the inflammatory cytokines, IL-1beta and TNF-alpha, was reduced significantly in the sRAGE-treated islets, compared with vehicle-treated animals. In addition, expression of IL-10 increased significantly in sRAGE-treated mice islets, along with increased TGF-beta, versus the vehicle-treated mice [38].

These key studies elucidated for the first time that the ligand–RAGE axis might play an important proximal role in the adaptive immune response. Studies to determine the precise links between RAGE and adaptive immunity in the context of dendritic cells and T lymphocytes should address these concepts.

Intriguingly, the premise that inflammation is a key component of mechanisms linked to insulin resistance suggests that roles for RAGE in the pathogenesis of type 2 diabetes should be addressed. The increased numbers of macrophages in obese, diabetic mice suggest links to the expression of TNF-alpha, iNOS and IL-6 in this setting [62]. Thus, given the expression of RAGE and its inflammatory ligands, S100/calgranulins and HMGB1 in macrophages, it is reasonable to test such concepts.

Blocking the ligand–receptor for advanced glycation end products axis: a therapeutic direction in diabetes and its complications

Stopping advanced glycation end products

Two distinct strategies are in various stages of development to either block AGE formation or to break AGE-related cross-linking in the tissues. A key agent studied in the context of preventing AGE formation has been aminoguanidine (or, pimagedine). When pimagedine was administered to 690 subjects with type 1 diabetes, nephropathy, and retinopathy, the estimated glomerular filtration rate progressed more slowly in the pimagedine-treated group, and the degree of proteinuria was significantly lower in the pimagedine-treated group [63]. However, this trial failed to meet statistical significance in the primary end point (doubling of serum creatinine). Nevertheless, studies using pimagedine were the first to support the AGE hypothesis and its role in diabetic complications in human subjects, even if based on changes in secondary end points.

The next level of anti-AGE strategies involves the AGE cross-link breakers. The prototypic agent, ALT-711, has already been tested in human clinical trials in nondiabetic subjects. In aging, increased cross-linking secondary to AGE effects occur. In human aged subjects, after 56 days treatment, ALT-711 resulted in improved total arterial compliance [64,65]. In addition, newer agents, such as pyridoxamine, an inhibitor of advanced glycation reactions, are in active clinical development, based on their efficacy in preclinical models of diabetes [66].

Lipid-soluble thiamine derivatives have been tested, based on the hypothesis of Brownlee and colleagues that glucose triggers three major pathways of hyperglycemic damage in the tissues (hexosamine, AGE formation, and diacylglycerol pathways), largely through generation of oxidative stress by way of mitochondrial pathways [67]. Long-term administration of benfotiamine resulted in decreased vascular abnormalities in the retina, and attenuated activation of NF-kB [67]. Further, other studies extended these findings to nephropathy; administration of either thiamine or benfotiamine to diabetic rats attenuated albuminuria [68]. These studies, a test of the concept of the glucose-triggered common pathway model of diabetic complications, provide potential new avenues for therapy in human subjects with diabetes. Large-scale clinical trials are needed to test these concepts fully.

Recent studies suggest that when food is exposed to high temperature conditions, AGEs form, resulting in the development of high-AGE diets. When human subjects consumed high- versus low-AGE food, inflammatory mediators were reduced [69]. In other studies, restriction of dietary glycotoxins reduced excess levels of AGEs in human subjects with renal failure [70].

Blockade of receptor for advanced glycation end products

Initial studies in animal models of diabetes and its complications have shown the efficacy of sRAGE. The studies using homozygous RAGE null mice strongly support the premise that the chief target of sRAGE is RAGE. In addition, in a number of studies, blocking antibodies to the receptor revealed effects identical to those from the administration of sRAGE. For example, in murine models of delayed type hypersensitivity and restenosis consequent to acute endothelial denudation, administration of $F(ab')_2$ fragments of anti-RAGE IgG exerted benefit in vivo, compared with such fragments prepared from nonimmune IgG [28,62]. Taken together, such studies suggest that administration of RAGE antagonists might be beneficial; clinical trials to address these concepts are on the horizon.

Summary

Although the RAGE axis and its blockade have yet to be tested in clinical trials, studies linking RAGE expression and levels of plasma sRAGE to human diabetes and cardiovascular disease suggest that this axis is probably relevant to the complications of hyperglycemia and inflammation. In perturbed vasculature, stresses induced by stimuli such as hyperlipidemia, physical injury, infection, or hyperglycemia may lead to upregulation of RAGE, thereby stimulating endothelial upregulation of inflammatory molecules and the recruitment of S100/calgranulin and HMGB1-bearing activated inflammatory cells. S100/calgranulins and HMGB1 may be released by these inflammatory cells in the vasculature. Thus, inflammatory cells bearing S100/calgranulins and HMGB1 may contribute integrally to mechanisms that initiate and advance atherosclerosis and vascular perturbation. In cardiovascular disease, particularly that consequent to long-term diabetes, multiple hits contribute to the initiation and progression of atherosclerosis, and, in advanced stages, to ischemia-reperfusion events. Efforts to delineate the precise steps at which RAGE plays contributory roles are critical in the optimal design of clinical trials to test these concepts.

References

[1] Garcia MJ, McNamara PM, Gordon T, et al. Morbidity and mortality in diabetics in the Framingham population. Sixteen year follow-up. Diabetes 1974;23:105–11.

[2] Panzram G. Mortality and survival in type (non-insulin-dependent) diabetes mellitus. Diabetologia 1987;30:123–31.

[3] United Kingdom Prospective Diabetes Study Group. UKPDS 17. A nine-year update of a randomized, controlled trial on the effect of improved metabolic control on complications in non-insulin-dependent diabetes mellitus. Ann Intern Med 1996;124:136–45.

[4] Krolewski AS, Kosinski EJ, Warram JH, et al. Magnitude and determinants of coronary artery disease in juvenile-onset, insulin-dependent diabetes mellitus. Am J Cardiol 1987;59: 750–5.

[5] Brownlee M. Glycation products and the pathogenesis of diabetic complications. Diabetes Care 1992;15:1835–43.

[6] Brownlee M. Advanced glycation endproducts in diabetic complications. Curr Opin Endocrinol Diabetes 1996;3:291–7.

[7] Anderson MM, Requena JR, Crowley JR, et al. The myeloperoxidase system of human phagocytes generates Nepsilon-(carboxymethyl)lysine on proteins: a mechanism for producing advanced glycation endproducts at sites of inflammation. J Clin Invest 1999;104:103–13.

[8] Traverso N, Menini S, Maineri EP, et al. Malondialdehyde, a lipoperoxidation-derived aldehyde, can bring about secondary oxidative damage to proteins. J Gerontol Biol Sci Med Sci 2004;59:B890–5.

[9] Ikeda K, Higashi T, Sano H, et al. Carboxymethyllysine protein adduct is a major immunological epitope in proteins modified with AGEs of the Maillard reaction. Biochem 1996;35: 8075–83.

[10] Reddy S, Bichler J, Wells-Knecht K, et al. Carboxymethyllysine is a dominant AGE antigen in tissue proteins. Biochem 1995;34:10872–8.

[11] Schleicher E, Wagner E, Nerlic A. Increased accumulation of glycoxidation product carboxymethyllysine in human tissues in diabetes and aging. J Clin Invest 1997;99:457–68.

[12] Thornalley PJ. Cell activation by glycated proteins. AGE receptors, receptor recognition factors and functional classification of AGEs. Cell Mol Biol (Noisy-le-grand) 1998;44:1013–23.

[13] Schmidt AM, Vianna M, Gerlach M, et al. Isolation and characterization of binding proteins for advanced glycosylation endproducts from lung tissue which are present on the endothelial cell surface. J Biol Chem 1992;267:14987–97.

[14] Neeper M, Schmidt AM, Brett J, et al. Cloning and expression of RAGE: a cell surface receptor for advanced glycosylation end products of proteins. J Biol Chem 1992;267: 14998–5004.

[15] Miyata T, Hori O, Zhang JH, et al. The Receptor for Advanced Glycation Endproducts (RAGE) mediates the interaction of AGE-b2 Microglobulin with human mononuclear

phagocytes via an oxidant-sensitive pathway: implications for the pathogenesis of dialysis-related amyloidosis. J Clin Invest 1996;98:1088–94.

[16] Schmidt AM, Yan SD, Brett J, et al. Regulation of mononuclear phagocyte migration by cell surface binding proteins for advanced glycosylation endproducts. J Clin Invest 1993;92: 2155–68.

[17] Sakaguchi T, Yan SF, Yan SD, et al. Arterial restenosis: central role of RAGE- dependent neointimal expansion. J Clin Invest 2003;111:959–72.

[18] Schmidt AM, Hori O, Chen J, et al. Advanced glycation endproducts interacting with their endothelial receptor induce expression of vascular cell adhesion molecule-1 (VCAM-1): a potential mechanism for the accelerated vasculopathy of diabetes. J Clin Invest 1995;96: 1395–403.

[19] Owen WF Jr, Hou FF, Stuart RO, et al. b2-Microglobulin modified with Advanced Glycation End Products modulates collagen synthesis by human fibroblasts. Kidney Int 1998;53: 1365–73.

[20] Wautier MP, Chappey O, Corda S, et al. Activation of NADPH Oxidase by Advanced Glycation Endproducts (AGEs) links oxidant stress to altered gene expression via RAGE. Am J Physiol Endocrinol Metab 2001;280:E685–94.

[21] Yan SD, Schmidt AM, Anderson G, et al. Enhanced cellular oxidant stress by the interaction of advanced glycation endproducts with their receptors/binding proteins. J Biol Chem 1994; 269:9889–97.

[22] Lander HL, Tauras JM, Ogiste JS, et al. Activation of the Receptor for Advanced Glycation Endproducts triggers a MAP Kinase pathway regulated by oxidant stress. J Biol Chem 1997; 272:17810–4.

[23] Basta G, Lazzerini G, Del Turco S, et al. At least two distinct pathways generating reactive oxygen species mediate vascular cell adhesion molecule-1 induction by advanced glycation end products. Arterioscler Thromb Vasc Biol 2005;25:1401–7.

[24] Wautier JL, Paton RC, Wautier MP, et al. Increased adhesion of erythrocytes to endothelial cells in diabetes mellitus and its relation to vascular complications. N Engl J Med 1981;305: 237–42.

[25] Wautier JL, Wautier MP, Schmidt AM, et al. Advanced glycation end products (AGEs) on the surface of diabetic erythrocytes bind to the vessel wall via a specific receptor inducing oxidant stress in the vasculature: a link between surface-associated AGEs and diabetic complications. Proc Natl Acad Sci USA 1994;91:7742–6.

[26] Kislinger T, Fu C, Huber B, et al. Nε (carboxymethyl)lysine modifications of proteins are ligands for RAGE that activate cell signaling pathways and modulate gene expression. J Biol Chem 1999;274:31740–9.

[27] Donato R. S100: a multigenic family of calcium-modulated proteins of the EF-hand type with intracellular and extracellular functional roles. Int J Biochem Cell Biol 2001;33:637–68.

[28] Hofmann MA, Drury S, Fu C, et al. RAGE mediates a novel proinflammatory axis: a central cell surface receptor for S100/calgranulin polypeptides. Cell 1999;97:889–901.

[29] Arumugam T, Simeone DM, Schmidt AM, et al. S100P stimulates cell proliferation and survival via RAGE. J Biol Chem 2004;279:5059–65.

[30] Frosch M, Strey A, Vogl T, et al. Myeloid-related proteins 8 and 14 are specifically secreted during interaction of phagocytes and activated endothelium and are useful markers for monitoring disease activity in pauciarticular-onset juvenile rheumatoid arthritis. Arthritis Rheum 2000;43:628–37.

[31] Rammes A, Roth J, Goebeler M, et al. Myeloid related protein (MRP) 8 and MRP14, calcium-binding proteins of the S100 family, are secreted by activated monocytes via a novel, tubulin-dependent pathway. J Biol Chem 1997;272:9496–502.

[32] Rauvala H, Pihlaskari R. Isolation and some characteristics of an adhesive factor of brain that enhances neurite outgrowth in central neurons. J Biol Chem 1987;262:16625–35.

[33] Hori O, Brett J, Slattery T, et al. The Receptor for Advanced Glycation Endproducts (RAGE) is a cellular binding site for amphoterin: mediation of neurite outgrowth and co-

expression of RAGE and amphoterin in the developing nervous system. J Biol Chem 1995;
270:25752–61.

[34] Taguchi A, Blood DC, del Toro G, et al. Blockade of amphoterin/RAGE signalling suppresses tumor growth and metastases. Nature 2000;405:354–60.

[35] Wang H, Bloom O, Zhang M, et al. HMG-1 as a late mediator of endotoxin lethality in mice.
Science 1999;285:248–51.

[36] Hofmann MA, Drury S, Hudson BI, et al. RAGE and arthritis: the G82S polymorphism amplifies the inflammatory response. Genes Immun 2002;3:123–35.

[37] Yan SSD, Wu ZY, Zhang HP, et al. Suppression of experimental autoimmune encephalomyelitis by selective blockade of encephalitogenic T-cell infiltration of the central nervous system. Nat Med 2003;9:287–93.

[38] Chen Y, Yan SS, Colgan J, et al. Blockade of late stages of autoimmune diabetes by inhibition of the receptor for advanced glycation end products. J Immunol 2004;173:
1399–405.

[39] Liliensiek B, Weigand MA, Bierhaus A, et al. Receptor for advanced glycation endproducts
(RAGE) regulates sepsis but not the adaptive immune response. J Clin Invest 2004;113:
1641–50.

[40] Kislinger T, Tanji N, Wendt T, et al. RAGE mediates inflammation and enhanced expression of tissue factor in the vasculature of diabetic apolipoprotein E null mice. Arterio
Thromb Vasc Biol 2001;21:905–10.

[41] Kosaki A, Hasegawa T, Kimura T, et al. Increased plasma S100A12 (EN-RAGE) levels in
patients with type 2 diabetes. J Clin Endocrinol Metab 2004;89:5423–8.

[42] Kalinina N, Agrotis A, Antropova Y, et al. Increased expression of the DNA binding cytokine HMGB1 in human atherosclerotic lesions: role of activated macrophages and cytokines. Arterioscler Thromb Vasc Biol 2004;24:2320–5.

[43] Yan SD, Zhu H, Golabek A, et al. Receptor-dependent cell stress and amyloid accumulation
in systemic amyloidosis. Nat Med 2000;6:643–51.

[44] Yan SD, Chen X, Fu J, et al. RAGE and amyloid-b peptide neurotoxicity in Alzheimer's disease. Nature 1996;382:685–91.

[45] Chavakis T, Bierhaus A, Al-Fakhri N, et al. The Pattern Recognition Receptor (RAGE) is
a counterreceptor for leukocyte integrins: a novel pathway for inflammatory cell recruitment. J Exp Med 2003;198:1507–15.

[46] Cipollone F, Iezzi A, Fazia M, et al. The Receptor RAGE as a progression factor amplifying
arachidonate-dependent inflammatory and proteolytic response in human atherosclerotic
plaques: role of glycemic control. Circulation 2003;108:1070–7.

[47] Falcone C, Emanuele E, D'Angelo A, et al. Plasma levels of soluble receptor for advanced
glycation endproducts and coronary artery disease in nondiabetic men. Arterioscler Thromb
Vasc Biol 2005;25:1032–7.

[48] Geroldi D, Falcone C, Emanuele E, et al. Decreased plasma levels of soluble receptor for advanced glycation endproducts in patients with essential hypertension. J Hypertens 2005;23:
1725–9.

[49] Katakami N, Matsuhisa M, Kaneto H, et al. Decreased endogenous secretory advanced glycation receptor in type 1 diabetic patients: its possible association with diabetic vascular complications. Diabetes Care 2005;28:2716–21.

[50] Koyama H, Shoji T, Yokoyama H, et al. Plasma level of endogenous secretory RAGE is associated with components of the metabolic syndrome and atherosclerosis. Arterioscler
Thromb Vasc Biol 2005;25:2587–93.

[51] Forbes JM, Thorpe SR, Thallas-Bonke V, et al. Modulation of soluble receptor for advanced
glycation endproducts by angiotensin-converting enzyme-1 inhibition in diabetic nephropathy. J Am Soc Nephrol 2005;16:2363–72.

[52] Petersson-Fernholm K, Forsblom C, Hudson BI, et al. The functional -374 T/A RAGE gene
polymorphism is associated with proteinuria and cardiovascular disease in type 1 diabetic
patients. Diabetes 2003;52:891–4.

[53] Falcone C, Campo I, Emanuele E, et al. Relationship between the-374 T/A RAGE gene polymorphism and angiographic coronary artery disease. Int J Mol Med 2004;14:1061–4.

[54] Falcone C, Campo I, Emanuele E, et al. -374 T/A polymorphism of the RAGE gene promoter in relation to severity of coronary atherosclerosis. Clin Chim Acta 2005;354:111–6.

[55] Hudson BI, Stickland MH, Futers TS, et al. Study of the -429T/C and -374T/A receptor for advanced glycation end products polymorphisms in diabetic and nondiabetic subjects with macrovascular disease. Diabetes Care 2001;24:2004.

[56] Kirbis J, Milutinovic A, Steblovnik K, et al. The -429 T/C and -374 T/A gene polymorphisms of the receptor for advanced glycation endproducts gene (RAGE) are not risk factors for coronary artery disease in Slovene population with type 2 diabetes. Coll Antropol 2004;28: 611–6.

[57] Hofmann MA, Yang Q, Harja E, et al. The RAGE Gly82Ser polymorphism is not associated with cardiovascular disease in the Framingham offspring study. Atherosclerosis 2005;182: 301–5.

[58] Park L, Raman KG, Lee KJ, et al. Suppression of accelerated diabetic atherosclerosis by soluble Receptor for AGE (sRAGE). Nat Med 1998;4:1025–31.

[59] Bucciarelli LG, Wendt T, Qu W, et al. RAGE blockade stabilizes established atherosclerosis in diabetic apolipoprotein E null mice. Circulation 2002;106:2827–35.

[60] Wendt T, Harja E, Bucciarelli L, et al. RAGE modulates vascular inflammation and atherosclerosis in a murine model of type 2 diabetes. Atherosclerosis 2005;(Jul):30 [epub ahead of print].

[61] Zhou Z, Wang K, Penn MS, et al. Receptor for AGE (RAGE) mediates neointimal formation in response to arterial injury. Circulation 2003;107:2238–43.

[62] Weisberg SP, McCann D, Desai M, et al. Obesity is associated with macrophage accumulation in adipose tissue. J Clin Invest 2003;112:1796–808.

[63] Bolton WK, Cattran DC, Williams ME, et al. ACTION I Investigator Group. Randomized trial of an inhibitor of formation of advanced glycation end products in diabetic nephropathy. Am J Pathol 2004;24:32–40.

[64] Kass DA, Shapiro EP, Kawaguchi M, et al. Improved arterial compliance by a novel advanced glycation endproduct crosslink breaker. Circulation 2001;104:1464–70.

[65] Susic D, Varagic J, Ahn J, et al. Cross link breakers: a new approach to cardiovascular therapy. Curr Opin Cardiol 2004;19:336–40.

[66] Onorato JM, Jenkins AJ, Thorpe SR, et al. Pyridoxamine, an inhibitor of advanced glycation reactions, also inhibits advanced lipoxidation reactions. Mechanism of action of pyridoxamine. J Biol Chem 2000;275:21177–84.

[67] Hammes HP, Du X, Edelstein D, et al. Benfotiamine blocks three major pathways of hyperglycemic damage and prevents experimental diabetic retinopathy. Nat Med 2003;9:294–9.

[68] Babaei-Jadidi R, Karachalias N, Ahmed N, et al. Prevention of incipient diabetic nephropathy by high-dose thiamine and benfotiamine. Diabetes 2003;52:2110–20.

[69] Vlassara H, Cai W, Crandall J, et al. Inflammatory mediators are induced by dietary glycotoxins, a major risk factor for diabetic angiopathy. Proc Natl Acad Sci USA 2003;99: 15596–601.

[70] Uribarri J, Peppa M, Cai W, et al. Restriction of dietary glycotoxins reduces excessive advanced glycation endproducts in renal failure patients. J Am Soc Nephrol 2003;14:728–31.

ELSEVIER
SAUNDERS

Endocrinol Metab Clin N Am
35 (2006) 525–549

ENDOCRINOLOGY
AND METABOLISM
CLINICS
OF NORTH AMERICA

Molecular and Signaling Mechanisms of Atherosclerosis in Insulin Resistance

Eric A. Schwartz, PhD[a], Peter D. Reaven, MD[b],*

[a]Division of Research, Carl T. Hayden VA Medical Center, 650 East Indian School Road,
Phoenix, AZ 85012, USA
[b]Division of Endocrinology, Carl T. Hayden VA Medical Center,
650 East Indian School Road, Phoenix, AZ 85012, USA

It has long been appreciated that atherosclerosis is accelerated and the incidence of cardiovascular disease (CVD) is higher in individuals with insulin resistance or type 2 diabetes mellitus [1,2]. Although it is now clear that numerous risk factors, such as hyperglycemia, hyperinsulinemia, dyslipidemia, and hypertension cluster in those with insulin resistance [3], how these factors accelerate atherosclerosis and increase CVD in these conditions of abnormal glucose metabolism has remained a mystery. In fact, as recently as 1992, the late Edwin Bierman acknowledged in his Duff Lecture "Atherogenesis in Diabetes" [4] that the underlying mechanisms of atherogenesis in this group of individuals could only be represented by a simple black box. Although his elegant summary of this field shed light on many of the potential risk factors in diabetes (eg, alterations in lipoprotein size and composition) within the black box that contribute to atherosclerosis, the signal pathways by which these factors promoted atherogenesis in vascular wall cells remained undefined.

In recent years it has become clear that atherosclerosis is a chronic inflammatory condition [5], characterized by influx of inflammatory cells into the vessel wall, and their production of bioactive proinflammatory factors. Once activated by products of these inflammatory cells (or other stimuli), vascular cells can further contribute to the inflammation by secreting many additional cytokines, eventually leading to a chronic self-propagating inflammatory process. Although the exact set of events initiating this vascular inflammation are unknown, it is quite clear that modification of all lipoproteins, whether by oxidative stress, aggregation, enzymatic activity,

* Corresponding author.
E-mail address: Peter.Reaven@va.gov (P.D. Reaven).

incorporation of acute phase inflammatory proteins, or addition of alde-hydes (such as glucose), greatly increases the accumulation and inflamma-tory potential of ApoB-containing lipoproteins [6,7] and decreases the anti-inflammatory properties of high-density lipoproteins (HDL). Thus, both lipoproteins (their entry, retention, and subsequent modification) and vascular inflammation play critical roles in the formation of the typical lipid rich atherosclerotic plaques in humans.

Numerous studies have demonstrated that both specific tissue inflamma-tion (eg, in adipose and hepatic tissue) and systemic inflammation are in-creased in insulin resistance [8–12] and may contribute to accelerated development of vascular diseases. For example, adipose tissue is a major producer of a variety of pro-inflammatory factors (adipokines), such as tumor necrosis factor alpha (TNFα), monocyte chemotactic protein (MCP)-1, interleukin (IL)-1β, IL-6, and plasminogen activator inhibitor (PAI)-1 [13,14]. Not surprisingly therefore, many of these factors are in-creased with obesity. There is increasing in vivo evidence that these adipo-kines act not only locally in a paracrine fashion to induce insulin resistance in surrounding adipose tissue but also act on distant tissues, such as skeletal muscle, to reduce systemic glucose uptake [9,15,16] and on hepatic tissue to stimulate C-reactive protein (CRP) and other acute phase response factors. In vitro and animal studies have also suggested that several of these systemic markers of inflammation and acute phase proteins themselves may also pro-mote inflammation and vascular cell injury [17–20]. Consistent with this po-tential role in vascular tissue, prospective studies in large cohorts have consistently demonstrated that many of these same factors, such as CRP, are independent predictors of atherosclerosis and CVD events [21–23].

An additional source of systemic inflammation may be insulin resis-tance and the compensatory hyperinsulinemia necessary to regulate glu-cose levels. Several investigators have demonstrated that systemic markers of inflammation increase with increasing parameters of the insu-lin resistance syndrome [24–26] and are higher in diabetic subjects with abnormalities predominantly in insulin resistance rather than in those with abnormalities in insulin secretion [27]. Consistent with this, we have shown that insulin resistance is associated with elevated levels of CRP [28] and decreased levels of adiponectin [29], independent of obesity [28,29]. Moreover, infusion of insulin in humans is associated with in-creases in inflammatory factors such as leptin [30] and declines in the anti-inflammatory factor adiponectin [31]. Thus, multiple lines of evidence support the concept that there is a close and potentially mutually rein-forcing relationship between obesity, inflammation, and insulin resistance (Fig. 1).

It is currently believed that the combination of genetic predisposition, nu-trient excess, and decreased physical activity contribute to the triad of obe-sity, insulin resistance, and inflammation. Although substantial controversy still exists as to the exact sequence of the development of these

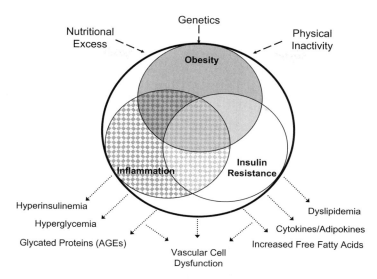

Fig. 1. Factors associated with insulin resistance contribute to vascular damage. A combination of nutrient excess, genetic predisposition, and lack of physical activity contribute to the pathophysiological triad of obesity, insulin resistance, and chronic inflammation. These three mutually reinforcing conditions induce numerous metabolic abnormalities including hyperinsulinemia, hyperglycemia, dyslipidemia, elevated plasma free fatty acids, increased inflammatory cytokines and adipokines, and increased formation of advanced glycation end products (AGEs). These factors in turn contribute to the increased development of atherosclerosis among individuals with insulin resistance (see Fig. 2).

abnormalities, it seems clear that they are closely linked, and have overlapping effects. One major consequence of this pathophysiological triad is the appearance of a broad variety of metabolic abnormalities, such as hyperinsulinemia, hyperglycemia and advanced glycation end products (AGEs), altered levels of cytokines and adipokines, elevated free fatty acids (FFAs), and dyslipidemia (see Fig. 1).

The potential of many of these metabolic abnormalities to enhance atherogenesis has been well characterized in numerous other publications, and several factors will be discussed in detail elsewhere in this issue. Therefore, the focus of this article will be on reviewing the current understanding of several cell signaling pathways (illustrated in a simplified form in Fig. 2) that may induce the vascular pathology, atherogenesis, and plaque rupture that occur more commonly in insulin resistance. Understanding these key pathways not only sheds further light into the "black box" of mechanisms of atherosclerosis and CVD in insulin resistance or type 2 diabetes, but may provide new insights into strategies to more effectively attenuate the consequences of the diverse array of cardiovascular risk factors associated with these conditions.

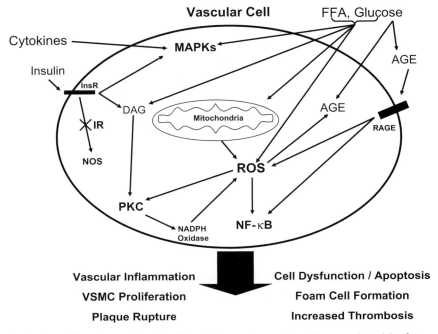

Fig. 2. Several key intracellular signaling pathways in vascular cells are activated by factors associated with insulin resistance. Pathways of vascular cell dysfunction may be activated by factors produced by obesity, insulin resistance, and vascular inflammation (Fig. 1). In vascular cells, the binding of insulin to the insulin receptor (InsR) induces intracellular signal cascades such as activation of nitric oxide synthase (NOS) and mitogen-activated protein kinases (MAPKs). In the setting of insulin resistance (IR), some signal cascades are attenuated (indicated by X), while others such as the MAPKs remain responsive to stimulation by insulin. Since insulin resistance leads to compensatory hyperinsulinemia, the MAPK pathways become excessively stimulated. Other risk factors present in the setting of insulin resistance include increased levels of inflammatory cytokines, elevated plasma free fatty acid (FFA) levels, and hyperglycemia; each of these factors can induce various intracellular signaling cascades. Both elevated FFA and hyperglycemia can cause nutrient overload of mitochondria, increase diacylglycerol (DAG) formation (causing activation of protein kinase C [PKC] and NADPH oxidase), and can also activate MAPKs. In addition, hyperglycemia leads to production of advanced glycation end products (AGE), which can not only result in intracellular protein damage but can also activate the AGE receptor (RAGE). Many of these activated signaling pathways result in the production of reactive oxygen species (ROS), which activate numerous mechanisms of vascular dysfunction. Among these is nuclear factor kappa B (NF-κB), a ROS-sensitive transcription factor that serves as a "master switch" of inflammation. Excessive amounts of ROS and AGE, as well as inappropriate activation of NF-κB, MAPK, and PKC results in altered gene transcription, leading to chronic vascular wall inflammation, cell dysfunction and apoptosis, vascular smooth muscle cell (VSMC) proliferation, infiltration of inflammatory cells into vascular tissue, formation of lipid-laden foam cells, weakening and rupture of the fibrous cap of atherosclerotic lesions, and hypercoagulability. These vascular abnormalities underlie the increased risk of cardiovascular disease in the setting of insulin resistance. Arrows indicate direction of signal/activation cascades; X indicates attenuation of signaling.

Nuclear factor kappa B: the inflammation master switch

Transcription factors of nuclear factor kappa B (NF-κB) family are central integrators of pro-inflammatory signals and master regulators of genes involved in inflammation, innate immunity, and atherosclerosis. This family comprises five known transcription factors: RelA (p65); RelB; c-Rel; NF-κB1 (p50); and NF-κB2 (p100, which is post-translationally processed to active p52), which all share a specific Rel homology domain that allows their dimerization, nuclear translocation, and DNA binding. Complexes of various combinations of these proteins are held in an inactive state in the cytoplasm of quiescent cells by inhibitory molecules known as IκB proteins. A major pathway of NF-κB activation is through stimulation of the membrane-associated inhibitor of kappa-B kinase (IKK) enzyme complex that promotes IκB protein phosphorylation, ubiquitination, and proteasomal degradation [32]. These events release NF-κB (eg, the p50/p65 complex), which then translocates into the nucleus where it mediates the transcription of a large number of target genes, including a multitude of pro-inflammatory genes [33].

It is well recognized that pro-inflammatory cytokines are important activators of the IKK/NF-κB pathway [33,34]. However, a variety of bacterial cell wall and viral products, double-stranded RNA, and mitogens can also indirectly induce activation of NF-κB [35,36]. Many of these factors activate the Toll-like receptors (TLR), a large and important family of surface and intracellular receptors that act as critical gatekeepers of the innate immune response. Stimulation of the TLR pathway leads to activation of NF-κB, which further propagates the host inflammation reaction. Although the TLR pathway appears to have originated as a protective mechanism against common bacterial and viral infections, when persistently activated at a low level it promotes chronic inflammation and may contribute to both insulin resistance and CVD.

Of great relevance are recent studies suggesting that several common features of obesity or insulin resistance, such as adipose, skeletal, and hepatic tissue inflammation; elevated levels of FFAs; hyperglycemia; and AGEs can contribute to activation of NF-κB [8,9,37–40]. In some cases, these factors generate increased amounts of reactive oxygen species (ROS), which are potent stimulators of NF-κB [41] (Fig. 2). However, in other instances, products of excess nutrition such as elevated levels of FFAs (or their increased flux into tissue) may activate the TLR pathway and lead to induction of the NF-κB program of cell inflammation. For example, certain saturated fatty acids, including palmitic acid (which accounts for up to 30% of the total plasma fatty acids) appear to be effective activators of the TLRs [42]. These events may be exacerbated in insulin-resistant individuals, where exaggerated postprandial rises in these factors can increase ROS formation or NF-κB activation and inflammation [43,44]. For example, meals containing either glucose or fat lead to generation of oxidative stress,

NF-κB activation, and inflammation [45]. A mixed meal containing a combination of these nutrients leads to even greater systemic inflammation than either alone [45]. These studies suggest that both the recurrent short-term insult of overeating, as well as the long-term consequences of overnutrition (ie, obesity) can contribute to NF-κB activation and systemic and vascular inflammation.

Consequences of nuclear factor kappa B activation

Fig. 3 includes a partial list of gene products that are driven by NF-κB activation. This central role of NF-κB in regulating the production of a wide variety of inflammatory proteins suggests that it is a critical integrator of pro-inflammatory signals and a master regulator of genes involved in inflammation, innate immunity, and atherosclerosis. Indeed, many of the pro-inflammatory gene products regulated by NF-κB have been linked to insulin resistance and type 2 diabetes [10,11,46–55]. Moreover, most of the mediators (cytokines, chemokines, receptors, surface adhesion molecules, and so forth) shown in Fig. 3 are also key players in vascular inflammation and atherogenesis [33,34]. For example, NF-κB is an important regulator of the factors required to induce monocyte chemotaxis, adhesion to endothelial cells, diapedesis into the intima of the arterial wall, and differentiation into macrophages. Similarly, NF-κB appears to control the global pro-inflammatory response of endothelial cells to various cytokines, such as TNFα [34],

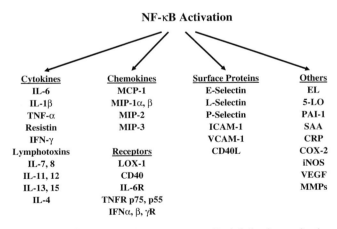

Fig. 3. Numerous pro-inflammatory genes are transcribed following activation of nuclear factor kappa B (NF-κB). NF-κB is a transcription factor that regulates much of the activity involved in cellular inflammation. Among the genes regulated by NF-κB are pro-inflammatory cytokines and chemokines (as well as receptors to many of these factors), surface proteins that modulate cell-cell inflammatory reactions, and numerous other proteins involved in inflammation, coagulation, vascular cell proliferation, angiogenesis, and the thinning and rupture of the fibrous cap of atherosclerotic plaques.

and also regulates vascular cell prothrombotic potential [56]. Although more controversial, there is evidence that vascular smooth muscle (VSMC) cell proliferation is enhanced by NF-κB activation and is attenuated by inhibitors of NF-κB [33,57,58]. This is supported by studies of animal vascular injury models, which show that NF-κB inhibition by NF-κB decoys or drug-eluting stents reduces neointimal formation [59–61]. Furthermore, NF-κB activation has been documented in human atherosclerotic plaques in macrophages, endothelial cells, and smooth cells. Therefore, it seems probable that NF-κB orchestrates the transcription of a constellation of genes that not only mediate obesity-induced insulin resistance [9,62] but also enhance atherosclerosis and CVD risk in insulin-resistant individuals. Despite the plethora of in vitro data to suggest that inhibition of NF-κB might slow atherosclerosis, this has been more difficult to demonstrate in animal models. Whereas deletion of NF-κB (p50 subunit) from hematopoietic cells decreased atherosclerosis [63] in mice, deletion of IκB kinase 2, one of the key stimulators of NF-κB in macrophage cells, actually increased atherosclerosis [64]. Tissue-specific deletions of IKKβ in mice had different effects depending on the tissue in which the enzyme was deleted: deletion of IKKβ from hepatocytes caused insulin resistance, whereas deletion of IKKβ from cells of myeloid lineage protected the mice from insulin resistance [65]. Clearly, the role of this transcription factor in atherosclerosis is complex, and (not surprisingly for such a critical regulator of inflammation and immunity) it has been demonstrated that NF-κB not only self-regulates its activity, but in certain situations also may promote resolution of inflammation [66].

Mitogen-activated protein kinases: mediators of cell growth and inflammation

Compensatory hyperinsulinemia frequently occurs in the insulin-resistant individual before hyperglycemia becomes evident [67]. Insulin levels must rise even higher during the postprandial period in these individuals to drive uptake and storage of their dietary glucose [68]. Normally, insulin engages its receptor and stimulates glucose uptake in adipose and skeletal tissue. The activated insulin receptor undergoes tyrosine autophosphorylation, allowing it to also phosphorylate insulin receptor substrate (IRS) proteins on tyrosine residues. Tyrosine phosphorylated IRS proteins initiate a cascade of intermediate kinase events that eventually drive translocation of the glucose transporter Glut4 to the cell surface [69]. In vascular wall endothelial cells, this pathway activates endothelial nitric oxide (NO) synthase, which promotes vasodilation, and reduces inflammation, platelet aggregation, and smooth muscle cell proliferation [70]. In contrast, a major action of insulin on VSMC is to cause mitogen-activated protein kinase (MAPK) activation, which leads to cell growth and proliferation, and PAI-1 production [71].

In the setting of insulin resistance, activation of several (but importantly not all) insulin-mediated signaling pathways are attenuated. For example, while muscle and adipose tissue Glut4 translocation is impaired in the insulin-resistant individual, the kidney tends to remain sensitive to insulin [72], where it promotes increased angiotensin receptor expression [73], sodium retention [72], and hypertension [72]. There is also evidence that key signaling pathways are variably affected in the vasculature of insulin-resistant individuals [74]. For example, insulin is less effective in stimulating IRS-1-mediated pathways in endothelial cells [68], which results in reduced NO synthesis and in endothelial dysfunction [71] (as discussed elsewhere in this volume). In contrast, in VSMC, IRS-independent MAPK pathways are largely spared [75], and so are excessively activated by compensatory hyper-insulinemia (Fig. 2). Because insulin sensitivity is retained in many tissues and signal pathways in the individual with insulin resistance, hyperinsuli-nema in this setting may contribute to a number of vascular complications mediated by the MAPK pathways.

Nature of the mitogen-activated protein kinase

The MAPKs are serine/threonine kinases, and include p38 MAPK, p44 and p42 extracellular regulated kinases (also called Erk1 and 2), c-Jun N-terminal kinases (or JNK1-3 [76]), and big MAP kinase, or BMK1 [77]. Binding of a large number of growth factors, cytokines, and other mitogens to their receptors induces a sequential cascade of kinases leading to the phosphorylation of MAPKs. In addition to receptor-mediated activation, Erk1/2 and BMK1 can be activated by ROS-mediated mechanisms [78,79]. MAPKs are also known to be regulated by several metabolic abnor-malities present in insulin resistance such as hyperosmolarity (due to hyper-glycemia) [74], elevated plasma FFA levels [74], and advanced glycation end products (AGEs) [80].

Upon activation, the MAPKs phosphorylate a number of transcription factors including Elk-1 (Erk1/2); c-Jun and JunD (JNK); ATF-2 (JNK and p38); and MAPKAP-K2/3, MEF2C, and GAD153 (p38) [81]. If these transcription factors are activated inappropriately, a variety of potentially deleterious alterations in gene expression may ensue. For ex-ample, phosphorylation of c-Jun by JNK initiates transcription of the pro-inflammatory genes TNF-α, IL-2, E-selectin, and collagenase-1 [82]. Similarly, activation of Elk-1 by Erk1/2 induces transcription of pro-atherosclerotic genes such as PAI-1 [83] and lectin-like oxLDL receptor-1 [84], and the pro-inflammatory genes MCP-1 and IL-8 [85]; and activation of p38 induces cell growth, apoptosis, and COX-2 expression in VSMC [86–88]. Hyperglycemia-induced activation of BMK1 in the mesangial cells of the diabetic rat kidney is associated with the development of glomeru-lonephrosis, although the role of BMK1 in this process is not yet entirely clear [77].

Several vascular complications of insulin resistance
are mediated by mitogen-activated protein kinase pathways

Inappropriate activation of the MAPK pathways as a consequence of insulin resistance leads to vascular dysfunction primarily due to three effects: VSMC proliferation, enhanced thrombotic potential, and increased monocyte recruitment and foam cell formation. There is abundant clinical evidence of disregulated proliferation of VSMC and restenosis following endothelial injury during angioplasty and stent placement/expansion [89]. VSMC proliferation is regulated, in large part, by MAPK pathways [88,90] in the setting of insulin resistance. Insulin-induced MAPK activation in VSMC has only a weak proliferative effect by itself [71,91], but greatly potentiates the proliferative effects of other growth factors, such as platelet-derived growth factor B, present in the injured vascular wall [71,87,88]. Although the details of the involved pathways are still being investigated, both p38 and BMK1 appear to regulate VSMC proliferation [87].

Approximately 80% of patients with diabetes will die from a thrombus, most commonly occluding an atherosclerotic coronary artery [92]. Susceptibility of these individuals to thrombosis is presumably a consequence of enhanced platelet activation and recruitment, enhanced coagulation, or decreased fibrinolysis, all of which are features common to type 2 diabetes and insulin resistance [93]. Recent investigations have shown that activation of MAPKs can contribute to these hemostatic abnormalities. Erk1/2 activation in endothelial cells [71] and VSMC [83] in response to hyperinsulinemia and hyperglycemia induces PAI-1 secretion, which inhibits fibrinolysis [93]. Furthermore, tissue factor, which promotes platelet aggregation, degranulation, and thrombosis, is released from vascular cells in response to inflammatory cytokines [94] that are regulated, at least in part, by Erk1/2 in endothelial cells [85], and by p38 in monocytes [95]. Last, excessive stimulation of MAPKs results in serine phosphorylation of IRS proteins, which in turn attenuates insulin-mediated NO synthesis by endothelial cells [96] and impairs their capacity to inhibit platelet aggregation [93].

Recruitment and subsequent infiltration of monocytes into the vessel wall is a key process in the development and progression of atherosclerotic disease [84]. MAPKs, and particularly the JNK subfamily, mediate expression of pro-inflammatory cytokines and endothelial cell-monocyte adhesion molecules (such as TNF-α and E-Selectin, respectively) in endothelial cells [82], and to some extent in monocytes as well [95]. For example, monocyte secretion of IL-6 in response to hyperglycemia is modulated by p38 [95]. In addition, glucose-activated Erk1/2 signaling in both monocytes and endothelial cells increases expression of lectin-like oxLDL receptor in a p38-dependent manner [84]. Moreover, JNK2 is required for scavenger receptor-A-mediated lipid uptake by monocytes, a crucial step in foam cell formation and plaque progression [97]. Last, JNKs mediate expression of matrix metalloproteinases, which degrade collagen and cause thinning and rupture of the fibrous cap of the unstable atherosclerotic plaque [82]. Therefore, MAPK activation appears to be a critical step linking hyperglycemia and compensatory hyperinsulinemia to the progression of atherosclerosis.

In addition to participating in mechanisms of vascular damage, hyperinsulinemia- and hyperglycemia-induced MAPK activation actually worsens insulin resistance itself. MAPKs can phosphorylate IRS-1 and -2 on serine residues, which does not activate the IRS-mediated signal cascade, but impairs the ability of the protein to be tyrosine phosphorylated by the insulin receptor. Thus, MAPKs, and especially the JNK subfamily, down-regulate the ability of the insulin receptor to induce glucose uptake or NO synthesis [96,98,99]. This would, of course, result in greater insulin resistance and hyperglycemia, further stimulating other pathways of vascular injury (eg, PKC).

In summary, MAPK pathways appear to play significant roles in the development of cardiovascular complications associated with insulin resistance. These occur, in part, because hyperinsulinemia activates the insulin-sensitive MAPK pathways even when insulin-mediated glucose uptake and NO synthesis are inhibited [71,73]. Effects of inappropriate MAPK activation on the vasculature include endothelial dysfunction [71], increased prothrombotic activity [83], monocyte recruitment and foam cell formation [84], and smooth muscle cell proliferation [88,89]. In addition, MAPKs act in a feed-forward loop to further increase insulin resistance [68]. It is worth cautioning, however, that MAPKs have diverse and essential functions in most tissues of the body. Consequently, while some MAPK antagonists have been used experimentally in the treatment of cancer [100–103], even highly specific therapeutic agents targeting a single MAPK can be risky candidate drugs, as other critical functions of these kinases would also be inhibited. More promising are efforts to identify specific pathways through which activated MAPKs induce diabetic complications, so that therapies can be designed to inhibit these deleterious pathways downstream of MAPK activation [104].

Protein kinase C: a family of enzymes with a multitude of effects on vascular cells

The protein kinase C (PKC) family of serine/threonine kinases comprises 11 isoforms in three subfamilies. PKC isoforms are classified into conventional, atypical, and novel subfamilies based on the stimuli that activate them. Conventional PKC isoforms (α, βI, βII, γ) are activated by both diacylglycerols (DAG) and calcium. Novel isoforms (δ, $\in$, η, θ) are activated by DAG but are insensitive to calcium. Last, atypical isoforms (ζ, ι, λ) are insensitive to both DAG and calcium, but appear to be regulated entirely by phosphatidylserine. All PKCs normally require phosphatidylserine to function, and so achieve a measure of substrate specificity since they remain inactive until they translocate from the cytoplasm to a phospholipid membrane [105]. Further substrate specificity is supplied by receptor of active C-kinase (RACK) proteins, which regulate which PKC isoforms will localize to which substrates [106].

Activation of protein kinase Cs in insulin resistance and type 2 diabetes mellitus

Several metabolic disturbances (such as chronic hyperglycemia, and elevated plasma FFA; Fig. 2) are exacerbated by nutritional excess, and in the insulin-resistant individual are further elevated during the postprandial period [107–109]. Cells exposed to elevated levels of glucose accumulate intracellular DAG [110] through nonenzymatic breakdown of glycolytic intermediates such as dihydroxy-acetone phosphate and glyceraldehyde-3-phosphate [111]. Hoffman and colleagues [110] also demonstrated that exposure of diabetic rat adipocytes to increased insulin levels augmented the DAG production from glucose, suggesting that an individual who is both hyperinsulinemic and hyperglycemic may have higher DAG levels (and thus, increased PKC activation) than in the presence of hyperglycemia alone. Last, AGEs (formed at a greater rate during hyperglycemia) can bind to the AGE receptor and activate PKC-mediated pathways [112,113].

The metabolism of dietary lipids can also stimulate production of DAG. During metabolism of a fat-containing meal, triglycerides are formed in the intestinal wall from two FFA molecules and a monoacylglycerol, and packaged into triglyceride-rich chylomicrons. The enzyme lipoprotein lipase (LPL) in the capillary beds hydrolyses the triglycerides in these particles to release FFA to the adipose and skeletal muscle tissue [114]. Because LPL has higher affinity for the sn-1 than the sn-2 and sn-3 positions of the glycerol backbone of the triglyceride [115,116] cleavage of sn-1 fatty acids generates DAG early in the LPL-mediated lipolytic cascade [116]. Much of this DAG is retained in lipoproteins [117], although some is transferred to cells by as-yet-unclear mechanisms. Certain synthetic DAG analogs like dioctanoylglycerol, however, are directly cell-permeable. In addition, phospholipid transfer protein has been shown to facilitate transfer of native DAG between lipoproteins [117].

FFAs can also activate PKCs by other mechanisms. For example, FFAs can induce phospholipase activation and generate DAG de novo from membrane phospholipids, activating both conventional and atypical PKCs [118]. Similarly, intracellular DAG levels can be raised by unsaturated FFA-mediated inhibition of DAG kinase, which normally breaks down excess DAG [119]. Arachidonic acid can activate phospholipase A2 through receptor-mediated mechanisms and activate atypical and novel PKCs [120]. Last, FFA can directly stimulate the DAG-binding site of PKCs, although with lower affinity than DAG itself [121–123].

As described elsewhere in this article, ROS are generated in increased amounts in insulin resistance and type 2 diabetes. ROS can activate PKC in several ways, as shown in Fig. 2 [124–127]. Peroxide can stimulate tyrosine phosphorylation of PKC-δ on amino acid 311, although the mechanism is unclear [125,128–131]. It has also been suggested that peroxide may directly damage the regulatory pseudosubstrate domain of the enzyme and produce a constitutively active PKC [125].

Consequences of protein kinase C activation in insulin resistance and type 2 diabetes mellitus

Because different PKC isoforms have widely divergent functions, a full discussion of the potential consequences of PKC activation in diabetes is beyond the scope of this review. However, George King and colleagues have published several excellent reviews on the roles of PKC in diabetic complications [118,132–137]. A partial listing of the potential proatherogenic consequences of PKC activation induced by hyperglycemia is presented in Table 1. It should also be noted that once activated, conventional and atypical PKC isoforms are depleted for time periods of 24 hours or more [134]. Therefore, the pathways inappropriately activated by PKC in the setting of insulin resistance will also be paradoxically refractory to stimulation in their normal, physiological roles [134]. The role of PKC in NADPH oxidase activation is covered in more detail below, as one example of the many potential vascular damage mechanisms mediated by PKC activation.

NADPH oxidase is an enzyme complex composed of multiple protein subunits. Its structure and activity were reviewed in detail by Sheppard and colleagues [138]. Briefly, the enzyme is activated when its cytosolic components are phosphorylated (mainly by PKC) resulting in a conformational change that exposes the binding domains of the p47^{phox} regulatory subunit.

Table 1
Protein kinase C-mediated pro-atherosclerotic effects of high glucose on vascular cells

Cell type	Effect	Isoforms	References
Monocyte	IL-6 production	α, β	[95]
Macrophage	LOX-1 expression	β	[84]
Endothelium	eNOS dysfunction	α, β, γ	[171]
Endothelium	ET-1 expression	β, δ	[172]
Endothelium	VCAM-1 expression	β	[173]
Endothelium	ICAM-1 expression	not determined	[174]
VSMC	proliferation	δ	[86]
VSMC	apoptosis	α, β, γ, ε, η, θ	[175]
Various	NADPH oxidase activity	α, β, γ, ε, η, θ	[176]

Abbreviations: eNOS, endothelial nitric oxide synthase; ET-1, endothelin-1, ICAM, intercellular adhesion molecule; IL, interleukin; LOX-1 lipoxygenase-1; NADPH, nicotinamide adenine dinucleotide phosphate; VCAM, vascular cell adlesion molecule.

Data from Rask-Madsen C, King GL. Proatherosclerotic mechanisms involving protein kinase C in diabetes and insulin resistance. Arterioscler Thromb Vasc Biol 2005;25(3):487–96; and Devaraj S, Venugopal SK, Singh U, Jialal I. Hyperglycemia induces monocytic release of interleukin-6 via induction of protein kinase c-{alpha} and -{beta}. Diabetes 2005;54(1):85–91.

This phosphorylation allows p47[phox] to recruit other subunits and translocate to the cell membrane. When fully assembled, the enzyme produces superoxide by catalyzing transfer of an electron from NADPH to oxygen [138]. Superoxide is not only a damaging chemical itself, but also is an important source for the synthesis of even more damaging ROS. As discussed in greater detail below, oxidative stress is a central player in the vascular pathologies of insulin resistance (see Fig. 2). Thus, by inducing NADPH oxidase-mediated ROS generation [139], PKC greatly amplifies its capacity to induce vascular damage [140].

Oxidative stress: a key link between pathways of cell activation and vascular disease

Oxidative stress plays a central role in the development of vascular complications associated with insulin resistance [70,112,134,140–145]. As discussed above, multiple intracellular pathways can lead to production of ROS, and many of these are excessively activated in the setting of insulin resistance and diabetes. Consistent with this concept, studies have demonstrated greater amounts of oxidative stress in plasma or mononuclear cells from subjects with insulin resistance or type 2 diabetes [146–148]. When present at elevated levels or in inappropriate locations, ROS can directly damage vascular cells through oxidative modification of proteins and DNA, and can indirectly enhance vascular inflammation and activation by inappropriately activating other cell-signaling pathways. This latter effect of ROS greatly amplifies both the number and severity of the deleterious downstream events they induce. For example, excessive generation of ROS leads to formation of oxidized LDL (low-density lipoprotein), which is a potent stimulator of chemokines, adhesion molecules, and scavenger receptors. Similarly, ROS are effective activators of the NF-κB inflammation pathway. Thus, ROS may be a critical mediator of vascular activation and injury in insulin resistance [142] (Fig. 2).

Sources of reactive oxygen species

There are several major sources of oxidative stress and ROS in insulin resistance or diabetes. Mitochondrial oxidative respiration may be the largest contributor of ROS in the basal state in most cell types [149]. To briefly review this pathway, mitochondria use an electron transport chain composed of enzyme complexes designated I to IV to produce ATP from the oxidation of nutrients (eg, glucose or fatty acids). Complexes I and II accept electrons from NADH and $FADH_2$ (generated by the metabolism of nutrients during the tricarboxylic acid cycle), respectively. During this process, these enzyme complexes pump hydrogen ions to the outside of the inner mitochondrial membrane, where they provide the voltage gradient that drives ATP synthase to convert ADP and phosphate into ATP. In the normal state,

Complex II passes its electrons through coenzyme Q to Complex III, and then on to Complex IV, and finally the electrons are transferred to hydrogen ions and molecular oxygen, which are then converted to water. However, in conditions where excess intracellular FFA or glucose develops (as may be seen in obese, insulin-resistant, or diabetic individuals), Complexes I and II expel larger numbers of hydrogen ions out of the inner mitochondrial membrane. If the voltage potential of the hydrogen ions outside the inner mitochondrial membrane exceeds the driving potential of Complex III, hydrogen ion transport (and therefore electron transport) across this complex ceases. When Complex III becomes unable to accept an electron, coenzyme Q will instead catalyze transfer of single electrons onto available oxygen molecules, leading to production of the ROS superoxide (which can also be converted to other forms of ROS [142,150]).

NADPH oxidase is another important source of ROS [149], as discussed above. This enzyme complex facilitates direct transfer of electrons from NADPH to oxygen to produce superoxide [139,140]. Although NADPH oxidase is not considered as great a source of ROS as that derived from mitochondrial oxidative respiration during nutritional excess, it is a dedicated oxidase, and when activated can rapidly increase the superoxide production by inflammatory cells many fold [140,149,151].

Hyperglycemia itself may increase ROS production through a number of additional pathways. For example, the non-enzymatic glycosylation reactions that produce AGEs in hyperglycemic individuals produce both superoxide and hydrogen peroxide as side-products [105]. In addition, the binding of AGEs to the AGE receptor, RAGE, activates NADPH oxidase and produces superoxide [112]. Furthermore, AGEs can induce DNA damage leading to overactivation of poly-(ADP-ribose) polymerase (PARP), a DNA repair enzyme that also inhibits activity of glyceraldehyde-3-phosphate dehydrogenase (GAPDH), a key enzyme in the metabolism of glucose [152]. When GAPDH activity is reduced, products proximal to this enzyme accumulate, and glyceraldehyde-3-phosphate is converted into DAG at an increased rate. This increase in DAG leads (as described above) to excessive activation of PKC and NADPH oxidase, resulting in increased generation of ROS [153].

Not only are pathways that increase ROS generation activated in insulin resistance and type 2 diabetes, but the antioxidant systems that normally protect cells from elevated levels of ROS excess are reduced. During sustained hyperglycemia, aldose reductase (which normally converts toxic intracellular aldehydes into inactive alcohols) converts excess glucose into sorbitol (the polyol pathway). This conversion depletes the cells of NADPH that would otherwise be used to regenerate reduced glutathione, one of the more important intracellular antioxidants. Additionally in insulin resistance, levels of asymmetric dimethyl arginine (an endogenous inhibitor of NO synthases) are increased and activity of dimethylarginine diaminohydrolase (the enzyme that degrades it) is decreased [154]. Together, these abnormalities decrease NO production. Under normal physiological conditions, NO has a number of vital functions: it acts as an antibacterial agent, a signaling molecule, and a scavenger of superoxide (depending on the cell type producing it). When NO production is low, scavenging of superoxide is decreased and levels of ROS are increased. Making matters worse, when inhibited from making NO by asymmetric dimethyl arginine, NO synthases retain activity as superoxide synthases and produce ROS [154]. Thus, both the increase in production of ROS and the decrease in antioxidant protection can contribute to vascular activation and damage in the insulin-resistant state.

Evidence of a central role for reactive oxygen species in vascular complications in insulin resistance

The important role of ROS in the pathogenesis of vascular complications in the setting of insulin resistance and diabetes has been well described in several recent reviews [142,147]. Support for the notion that ROS-mediated pathways within the vascular cell may predominate over those that are glycation-mediated comes in part from several clinical observations. Most nondiabetic insulin-resistant individuals do not experience marked daylong hyperglycemia (and therefore do not have greatly enhanced AGE formation) and yet they remain at increased risk of CVD [67]. This suggests glycation-mediated mechanisms cannot be the only factors underlying the vascular complications associated with insulin resistance. Moreover, it has been difficult to demonstrate that therapy that primarily lowers blood glucose is an effective modality to reduce CVD [155–157].

The importance of ROS results in part from their central location in the nexus of activation pathways within vascular cells, as is illustrated schematically in Fig. 2.

As described, multiple pathways of vascular cell activation, including those mediated via PKC [139], MAPK [158], and AGEs [105] lead to formation of ROS. Although it is clear that ROS can directly and indirectly contribute to structural and functional vascular abnormalities, ROS are also key activators of numerous intracellular signaling pathways related to vascular disease in insulin resistance (Fig. 2). For example, ROS can oxidatively modify the regulatory psuedosubstrate domain of PKC isoforms and produce a constitutively active PKC, causing aberrant signaling and gene transcription [125], and amplifying oxidative stress by activating NADPH oxidase [139]. Depletion of NO by ROS leads to endothelial dysfunction (including increases in vascular permeability, platelet and leukocyte adhesivity, and oxidative and nitrosative protein and DNA damage), loss of flow-mediated vasodilation, and proliferation of VSMC [70]. Reactive oxygen species are also well recognized as key activators of the "master switch" of cellular inflammation, NF-κB [159]. Moreover, as elegantly reviewed by Brownlee in his 2004 Banting Lecture [142], ROS, and especially superoxide produced by the mitochondrial electron transport chain, may be largely responsible for several pathways of glucose-mediated cell activation and injury. How does this occur? A critical step in the glycolytic pathway of glucose is the conversion of glyceraldehyde-3 phosphate to 1,3 disphosphoglycerate by the enzyme GAPDH. As noted above, excess superoxide can indirectly inhibit GAPDH activity. One consequence of this is elevated levels of all the glycolytic intermediates preceding 1,3 disphosphoglycerate, including glyceraldehyde-3 phosphate, fructose-6-phosphate, and glucose itself. Elevated intracellular levels of each of these precursors has been demonstrated to enhance flux through four major pathways responsible for hyperglycemic damage: (1) formation of AGEs; (2) activation of PKC; (3) activation of the hexosamine pathway; and (4) excessive formation of sorbitol [159]. In this fashion, excessive generation of ROS may be a unifying mechanism for many of the vascular complications of hyperglycemia.

Summary and clinical implications

In the past decade great progress has been made in understanding how molecular mechanisms that may enhance vascular disease are associated with insulin resistance. We now recognize that a number of the metabolic abnormalities present in insulin resistance, such as hyperglycemia and elevated plasma FFA, can stimulate one or more central pathways of vascular cell activation, inflammation, and injury, and that the involved signaling pathways (NF-κB, MAPK, PKC, and intracellular ROS formation) are frequently closely interconnected. Thus, initiation of a single pathway may activate others. In addition, there is a new appreciation that the responses of different tissues to stimuli may differ, and that cross talk between tissues is important in the development of chronic inflammatory conditions. Inflammation in hepatic and adipose tissue, for example, leads to the generation of a number of paracrine and hormone-like factors that reduce insulin signaling in some tissues (eg, skeletal muscle), and at the same time drive inflammation and atherogenesis (especially in the setting of dyslipidemia) in the vascular wall. These advances have led to the identification of several new risk factors and key vascular cell signal pathways within Bierman's "black box" of atherogenesis in individuals with insulin resistance and type 2 diabetes.

The recognition that multiple signaling pathways contribute to vascular cell pathology provides a new framework for understanding earlier, unexplained clinical findings. Although hyperglycemia is clearly an important direct and indirect stimulator of intracellular MAPK, PKC, and NF-κB, other factors (eg, elevated levels of FFAs, insulin, cytokines, and especially ROS) present in the prediabetes state can also drive these proatherogenic and prothrombotic pathways. For this reason, it is easy to understand why most studies have found that improving glycemic control alone, without correcting other metabolic abnormalities, does not reduce CVD in type 2 diabetes [155–157].

Identification of these important pathways of cell activation also provides new opportunities for prevention and intervention to reduce CVD. Since many of these pathways are activated by nutritional factors or their products, excess ingestion of carbohydrates or fats may directly or indirectly drive vascular cell activation in the short term. Moreover, chronic excess caloric intake that results in obesity and hepatic and adipose tissue inflammation is accompanied by insulin resistance and hyperinsulinemia, which, in turn, drives vascular inflammation. These interrelated events underscore the importance of nutritional education and weight loss in individuals at risk for diabetes and CVD. There is also great interest in developing pharmaceuticals that inhibit specific pathogenic vascular cell-signaling pathways. To this end, inhibitors of various PKC isoforms are already in development and have shown partial success in ameliorating microvascular disease in patients. Efforts are ongoing to assess their value in treating macrovascular disease. Although agents that inhibit NF-κB, a transcription factor that regulates so many genes, raises concerns, there is evidence that this could be a useful therapeutic approach. Vascular stents coated with NF-κB inhibitors have had success in limiting restenosis, and high-dose salicylates (which reduce IκBα phosphorylation by the IKK complex) have been found to lower blood glucose, increase insulin sensitivity, and decrease systemic inflammation [160]. In addition, thiazolidinediones provide a good example of how modulation of a single gene transcription factor (PPAR-γ) that has a broad range of metabolic effects, can prove clinically beneficial. Thiazolidinediones and other agents that increase insulin sensitivity also appear to improve several of the metabolic abnormalities (eg, dyslipidemia, hyperglycemia, elevated levels of cytokines, and increased plasma FFA levels) that initiate vascular cell activation and inflammation [161–163]. Several ongoing studies will soon provide results that will indicate whether these improvements in metabolic abnormalities translate into reduced CVD. Although initial trials of conventional antioxidant compounds such as vitamin E have not generally been successful in reducing CVD [164–167], there is hope that new catalytic antioxidant enzymes, such as a SOD/catalase mimetic [168–170] will be more effective in reducing the damaging effects of intracellular ROS. Finally, as we learn more about signaling pathways that contribute to vascular cell activation, it is likely that we will be better able to design therapies that selectively inhibit their harmful consequences.

References

[1] Pyorälä K, Laakso M, Uusitupa M. Diabetes and atherosclerosis: an epidemiologic view. Diabetes Metab Rev 1987;3:463–524.
[2] Kannel WB, McGee DL. Diabetes and cardiovascular disease. The Framingham study. JAMA 1979;241(19):2035–8.
[3] Reaven GM. Banting lecture 1988. Role of insulin resistance in human disease. Diabetes 1988;37(12):1595–607.
[4] Bierman EL. George Lyman Duff Memorial Lecture. Atherogenesis in diabetes. Arterioscler Thromb 1992;12:647–56.
[5] Ross R. Atherosclerosis is an inflammatory disease. Am Heart J 1999;138(5 Pt 2):S419–20.

 [6] Steinberg D, Parthasarathy S, Carew TE, et al. Beyond cholesterol modifications of low-density lipoprotein that increase its atherogenicity. N Engl J Med 1989;320:915–24.
 [7] Navab M, Berliner JA, Watson AD, et al. The Yin and Yang of oxidation in the development of the fatty streak. A review based on the 1994 George Lyman Duff Memorial Lecture. Arterioscler Thromb Vasc Biol 1996;16(7):831–42.
 [8] Shoelson SE, Lee J, Yuan M. Inflammation and the IKK beta/I kappa B/NF-kappa B axis in obesity- and diet-induced insulin resistance. Int J Obes Relat Metab Disord 2003; 27(Suppl 3):S49–52.
 [9] Cai D, Yuan M, Frantz DF, et al. Local and systemic insulin resistance resulting from hepatic activation of IKK-beta and NF-kappaB. Nat Med 2005;11(2):183–90.
[10] Pradhan AD, Manson JE, Rifai N, et al. C-Reactive protein, interleukin 6, and risk of developing type 2 diabetes mellitus. JAMA 2001;286(3):327–34.
[11] Festa A, D'Agostino R Jr, Howard G, et al. Chronic subclinical inflammation as part of the insulin resistance syndrome: the Insulin Resistance Atherosclerosis Study (IRAS). Circulation 2000;102(1):42–7.
[12] Yudkin JS, Juhan-Vague I, Hawe E, et al. Low-grade inflammation may play a role in the etiology of the metabolic syndrome in patients with coronary heart disease: the HIFMECH study. Metabolism 2004;53(7):852–7.
[13] Lau DC, Dhillon B, Yan H, et al. Adipokines: molecular links between obesity and atheroslcerosis. Am J Physiol Heart Circ Physiol 2005;288(5):H2031–41.
[14] Funahashi T, Nakamura T, Shimomura I, et al. Role of adipocytokines on the pathogenesis of atherosclerosis in visceral obesity. Intern Med 1999;38(2):202–6.
[15] Gabriely I, Ma XH, Yang XM, et al. Removal of visceral fat prevents insulin resistance and glucose intolerance of aging: an adipokine-mediated process? Diabetes 2002;51(10):2951–8.
[16] Havel PJ. Control of energy homeostasis and insulin action by adipocyte hormones: leptin, acylation stimulating protein, and adiponectin. Curr Opin Lipidol 2002;13(1):51–9.
[17] Libby P, Sukhova G, Lee RT, et al. Cytokines regulate vascular functions related to stability of the atherosclerotic plaque. J Cardiovasc Pharmacol 1995;25(Suppl 2):S9–12.
[18] Weyer C, Yudkin JS, Stehouwer CD, et al. Humoral markers of inflammation and endothelial dysfunction in relation to adiposity and in vivo insulin action in Pima Indians. Atherosclerosis 2002;161(1):233–42.
[19] Festa A, D'Agostino R Jr, Williams K, et al. The relation of body fat mass and distribution to markers of chronic inflammation. Int J Obes Relat Metab Disord 2001;25(10):1407–15.
[20] Ridker PM, Cushman M, Stampfer MJ, et al. Plasma concentration of C-reactive protein and risk of developing peripheral vascular disease. Circulation 1998;97(5):425–8.
[21] Ridker PM, Glynn RJ, Hennekens CH. C-reactive protein adds to the predictive value of total and HDL cholesterol in determining risk of first myocardial infarction. Circulation 1998;97(20):2007–11.
[22] Pradhan AD, Manson JE, Rossouw JE, et al. Inflammatory biomarkers, hormone replacement therapy, and incident coronary heart disease: prospective analysis from the Women's Health Initiative observational study. JAMA 2002;288(8):980–7.
[23] Ridker PM, Stampfer MJ, Rifai N. Novel risk factors for systemic atherosclerosis: a comparison of C-reactive protein, fibrinogen, homocysteine, lipoprotein(a), and standard cholesterol screening as predictors of peripheral arterial disease. JAMA 2001; 285(19):2481–5.
[24] Ford ES, Ajani UA, Mokdad AH. The metabolic syndrome and concentrations of C-reactive protein among US youth. Diabetes Care 2005;28(4):878–81.
[25] Ridker PM, Buring JE, Cook NR, et al. C-reactive protein, the metabolic syndrome, and risk of incident cardiovascular events: an 8-year follow-up of 14 719 initially healthy American women. Circulation 2003;107(3):391–7.
[26] Frohlich M, Imhof A, Berg G, et al. Association between C-reactive protein and features of the metabolic syndrome: a population-based study. Diabetes Care 2000;23(12):1835–9.

[27] Haffner SM. Metabolic syndrome, diabetes and coronary heart disease. Int J Clin Pract Suppl 2002;56(Suppl 132):31–7.

[28] McLaughlin T, Abbasi F, Lamendola C, et al. Differentiation between obesity and insulin resistance in the association with C-reactive protein. Circulation 2002;106(23): 2908–12.

[29] Abbasi F, Chu JW, Lamendola C, et al. Discrimination between obesity and insulin resistance in the relationship with adiponectin. Diabetes 2004;53(3):585–90.

[30] Saad MF, Khan A, Sharma A, et al. Physiological insulinemia acutely modulates plasma leptin. Diabetes 1998;47(4):544–9.

[31] Yu JG, Javorschi S, Hevener AL, et al. The effect of thiazolidinediones on plasma adiponectin levels in normal, obese, and type 2 diabetic subjects. Diabetes 2002; 51(10):2968–74.

[32] Collins T. Endothelial Nuclear Factor-kB and the Initiation of the Atherosclerosis Lesion. Lab Invest 1993;68(5):499–508.

[33] Thurberg BL, Collins T. The nuclear factor-kappa B/inhibitor of kappa B autoregulatory system and atherosclerosis. Curr Opin Lipidol 1998;9(5):387–96.

[34] Kempe S, Kestler H, Lasar A, et al. NF-kappaB controls the global pro-inflammatory response in endothelial cells: evidence for the regulation of a pro-atherogenic program. Nucleic Acids Res 2005;33(16):5308–19.

[35] Baeuerle PA, Baltimore D. NF-kappa B: ten years after. Cell 1996;87(1):13–20.

[36] Rothwarf DM, Karin M. The NF-kappa B activation pathway: a paradigm in information transfer from membrane to nucleus. Sci STKE 1999;1999(5) RE1.

[37] Aljada A, Mohanty P, Ghanim H, et al. Increase in intranuclear nuclear factor kappaB and decrease in inhibitor kappaB in mononuclear cells after a mixed meal: evidence for a proinflammatory effect. Am J Clin Nutr 2004;79(4):682–90.

[38] Dhindsa S, Tripathy D, Mohanty P, et al. Differential effects of glucose and alcohol on reactive oxygen species generation and intranuclear nuclear factor-kappaB in mononuclear cells. Metabolism 2004;53(3):330–4.

[39] Morigi M, Angioletti S, Imberti B, et al. Leukocyte-endothelial interaction is augmented by high glucose concentrations and hyperglycemia in a NF-kB-dependent fashion. J Clin Invest 1998;101:1905–15.

[40] Weigert C, Brodbeck K, Staiger H, et al. Palmitate, but not unsaturated fatty acids, induces the expression of interleukin-6 in human myotubes through proteasome-dependent activation of nuclear factor-kappaB. J Biol Chem 2004;279(23):23942–52.

[41] Kabe Y, Ando K, Hirao S, et al. Redox regulation of NF-kappaB activation: distinct redox regulation between the cytoplasm and the nucleus. Antioxid Redox Signal 2005;7(3–4): 395–403.

[42] Lee JY, Zhao L, Youn HS, et al. Saturated fatty acid activates but polyunsaturated fatty acid inhibits Toll-like receptor 2 dimerized with Toll-like receptor 6 or 1. J Biol Chem 2004;279(17):16971–9.

[43] Mohanty P, Hamouda W, Garg R, et al. Glucose challenge stimulates reactive oxygen species (ROS) generation by leucocytes. J Clin Endocrinol Metab 2000;85(8):2970–3.

[44] Mohanty P, Ghanim H, Hamouda W, et al. Both lipid and protein intakes stimulate increased generation of reactive oxygen species by polymorphonuclear leukocytes and mononuclear cells. Am J Clin Nutr 2002;75(4):767–72.

[45] Ceriello A, Taboga C, Tonutti L, et al. Evidence for an independent and cumulative effect of postprandial hypertriglyceridemia and hyperglycemia on endothelial dysfunction and oxidative stress generation: effects of short- and long-term simvastatin treatment. Circulation 2002;106(10):1211–8.

[46] Pickup JC, Crook MA. Is type II diabetes mellitus a disease of the innate immune system? Diabetologia 1998;41(10):1241–8.

[47] Hotamisligil GS, Spiegelman BM. Tumor necrosis factor alpha: a key component of the obesity-diabetes link. Diabetes 1994;43(11):1271–8.

[48] Duncan BB, Schmidt MI, Pankow JS, et al. Low-grade systemic inflammation and the development of type 2 diabetes: the atherosclerosis risk in communities study. Diabetes 2003; 52(7):1799–805.

[49] Festa A, D'Agostino R Jr, Tracy RP, et al. Elevated levels of acute-phase proteins and plasminogen activator inhibitor-1 predict the development of type 2 diabetes: the insulin resistance atherosclerosis study. Diabetes 2002;51(4):1131–7.

[50] Hotamisligil GS, Shargill NS, Spiegelman BM. Adipose expression of tumor necrosis factor-alpha: direct role in obesity-linked insulin resistance. Science 1993;259(5091):87–91.

[51] Inoue Y, Otsuka T, Niiro H, et al. Novel regulatory mechanisms of CD40-induced prostanoid synthesis by IL-4 and IL-10 in human monocytes. J Immunol 2004;172(4): 2147–54.

[52] Klover PJ, Zimmers TA, Koniaris LG, et al. Chronic exposure to interleukin-6 causes hepatic insulin resistance in mice. Diabetes 2003;52(11):2784–9.

[53] Perreault M, Marette A. Targeted disruption of inducible nitric oxide synthase protects against obesity-linked insulin resistance in muscle. Nat Med 2001;7(10):1138–43.

[54] Rui L, Yuan M, Frantz D, et al. SOCS-1 and SOCS-3 block insulin signaling by ubiquitin-mediated degradation of IRS1 and IRS2. J Biol Chem 2002;277(44):42394–8.

[55] Ventre J, Doebber T, Wu M, et al. Targeted disruption of the tumor necrosis factor-alpha gene: metabolic consequences in obese and nonobese mice. Diabetes 1997;46(9): 1526–31.

[56] Monaco C, Andreakos E, Kiriakidis S, et al. Canonical pathway of nuclear factor kappa B activation selectively regulates proinflammatory and prothrombotic responses in human atherosclerosis. Proc Natl Acad Sci U S A 2004;101(15):5634–9.

[57] De Martin R, Hoeth M, Hofer-Warbinek R, et al. The transcription factor NF-kappa B and the regulation of vascular cell function. Arterioscler Thromb Vasc Biol 2000;20(11): E83–8.

[58] Mehrhof FB, Schmidt-Ullrich R, Dietz R, et al. Regulation of vascular smooth muscle cell proliferation: role of NF-kappaB revisited. Circ Res 2005;96(9):958–64.

[59] Chen YX, Ma X, Whitman S, et al. Novel antiinflammatory vascular benefits of systemic and stent-based delivery of ethylisopropylamiloride. Circulation 2004;110(24):3721–6.

[60] Jun-Ichi S, Hiroshi I, Ryo G, et al. Initial clinical cases of the use of a NF-kappaB decoy at the site of coronary stenting for the prevention of restenosis. Circ J 2004;68(3):270–1.

[61] Zuckerbraun BS, McCloskey CA, Mahidhara RS, et al. Overexpression of mutated Ikappa-paBalpha inhibits vascular smooth muscle cell proliferation and intimal hyperplasia formation. J Vasc Surg 2003;38(4):812–9.

[62] Cai G, Cole SA, Tejero ME, et al. Pleiotropic effects of genes for insulin resistance on adiposity in baboons. Obes Res 2004;12(11):1766–72.

[63] Kanters E, Gijbels MJ, van der Made I, et al. Hematopoietic NF-kappaB1 deficiency results in small atherosclerotic lesions with an inflammatory phenotype. Blood 2004;103(3): 934–40.

[64] Kanters E, Pasparakis M, Gijbels MJ, et al. Inhibition of NF-kappaB activation in macrophages increases atherosclerosis in LDL receptor-deficient mice. J Clin Invest 2003;112(8): 1176–85.

[65] Arkan MC, Hevener AL, Greten FR, et al. IKK-beta links inflammation to obesity-induced insulin resistance. Nat Med 2005;11(2):191–8.

[66] Lawrence T, Gilroy DW, Colville-Nash PR, et al. Possible new role for NF-kappaB in the resolution of inflammation. Nat Med 2001;7(12):1291–7.

[67] Ramlo-Halsted BA, Edelman SV. The natural history of type 2 diabetes. Implications for clinical practice. Prim Care 1999;26(4):771–89.

[68] Krook A, Wallberg-Henriksson H, Zierath JR. Sending the signal: molecular mechanisms regulating glucose uptake. Med Sci Sports Exerc 2004;36(7):1212–7.

[69] Thong FS, Dugani CB, Klip A. Turning signals on and off: GLUT4 traffic in the insulin-signaling highway. Physiology (Bethesda) 2005;20:271–84.

[70] Hsueh WA, Quinones MJ. Role of endothelial dysfunction in insulin resistance. Am J Cardiol 2003;92(4A) 10J–7J.

[71] Hsueh WA, Law RE. Insulin signaling in the arterial wall. Am J Cardiol 1999;84(1A): 21J–4J.

[72] Catena C, Giacchetti G, Novello M, et al. Cellular mechanisms of insulin resistance in rats with fructose-induced hypertension. Am J Hypertens 2003;16(11 Pt 1):973–8.

[73] Hussain T. Renal angiotensin II receptors, hyperinsulinemia, and obesity. Clin Exp Hypertens 2003;25(7):395–403.

[74] Evans JL, Goldfine ID, Maddux BA, et al. Oxidative stress and stress-activated signaling pathways: a unifying hypothesis of type 2 diabetes. Endocr Rev 2002;23(5):599–622.

[75] Cusi K, Maezono K, Osman A, et al. Insulin resistance differentially affects the PI 3-kinase- and MAP kinase-mediated signaling in human muscle. J Clin Invest 2000;105(3): 311–20.

[76] Karin M, Gallagher E. From JNK to pay dirt: jun kinases, their biochemistry, physiology and clinical importance. IUBMB Life 2005;57(4–5):283–95.

[77] Suzaki Y, Yoshizumi M, Kagami S, et al. BMK1 is activated in glomeruli of diabetic rats and in mesangial cells by high glucose conditions. Kidney Int 2004;65(5):1749–60.

[78] Foncea R, Carvajal C, Almarza C, et al. Endothelial cell oxidative stress and signal transduction. Biol Res 2000;33(2):89–96.

[79] Greene EL, Velarde V, Jaffa AA. Role of reactive oxygen species in bradykinin-induced mitogen-activated protein kinase and c-fos induction in vascular cells. Hypertension 2000;35(4):942–7.

[80] Ishihara K, Tsutsumi K, Kawane S, et al. The receptor for advanced glycation end-products (RAGE) directly binds to ERK by a D-domain-like docking site. FEBS Lett 2003;550(1–3):107–13.

[81] Kaminska B. MAPK signalling pathways as molecular targets for anti-inflammatory therapy-from molecular mechanisms to therapeutic benefits. Biochim Biophys Acta 2005;1754: 253–62.

[82] Manning AM, Davis RJ. Targeting JNK for therapeutic benefit: from junk to gold? Nat Rev Drug Discov 2003;2(7):554–65.

[83] Suzuki M, Akimoto K, Hattori Y. Glucose upregulates plasminogen activator inhibitor-1 gene expression in vascular smooth muscle cells. Life Sci 2002;72(1):59–66.

[84] Li L, Sawamura T, Renier G. Glucose enhances human macrophage LOX-1 expression: role for LOX-1 in glucose-induced macrophage foam cell formation. Circ Res 2004; 94(7):892–901.

[85] Bowdish DM, Davidson DJ, Speert DP, et al. The human cationic peptide LL-37 induces activation of the extracellular signal-regulated kinase and p38 kinase pathways in primary human monocytes. J Immunol 2004;172(6):3758–65.

[86] Igarashi M, Wakasaki H, Takahara N, et al. Glucose or diabetes activates p38 mitogen-activated protein kinase via different pathways. J Clin Invest 1999;103(2):185–95.

[87] Zhao M, Liu Y, Bao M, et al. Vascular smooth muscle cell proliferation requires both p38 and BMK1 MAP kinases. Arch Biochem Biophys 2002;400(2):199–207.

[88] Yamaguchi H, Igarashi M, Hirata A, et al. Altered PDGF-BB-induced p38 MAP kinase activation in diabetic vascular smooth muscle cells: roles of protein kinase C-delta. Arterioscler Thromb Vasc Biol 2004;24(11):2095–101.

[89] Nishio K, Fukui T, Tsunoda F, et al. Insulin resistance as a predictor for restenosis after coronary stenting. Int J Cardiol 2005;103(2):128–34.

[90] Srivastava AK. High glucose-induced activation of protein kinase signaling pathways in vascular smooth muscle cells: a potential role in the pathogenesis of vascular dysfunction in diabetes (review). Int J Mol Med 2002;9(1):85–9.

[91] Igarashi M, Yamaguchi H, Hirata A, et al. Insulin activates p38 mitogen-activated protein (MAP) kinase via a MAP kinase kinase (MKK) 3/MKK 6 pathway in vascular smooth muscle cells. Eur J Clin Invest 2000;30(8):668–77.

[92] Aras R, Sowers JR, Arora R. The proinflammatory and hypercoagulable state of diabetes mellitus. Rev Cardiovasc Med 2005;6(2):84–97.

[93] Sobel BE, Schneider DJ. Platelet function, coagulopathy, and impaired fibrinolysis in diabetes. Cardiol Clin 2004;22(4):511–26.

[94] Szotowski B, Antoniak S, Poller W, et al. Procoagulant soluble tissue factor is released from endothelial cells in response to inflammatory cytokines. Circ Res 2005;96(12):1233–9.

[95] Devaraj S, Venugopal SK, Singh U, et al. Hyperglycemia induces monocytic release of interleukin-6 via induction of protein kinase c-{alpha} and -{beta}. Diabetes 2005;54(1): 85–91.

[96] Gual P, Gremeaux T, Gonzalez T, et al. MAP kinases and mTOR mediate insulin-induced phosphorylation of insulin receptor substrate-1 on serine residues 307, 612 and 632. Diabetologia 2003;46(11):1532–42.

[97] Sumara G, Belwal M, Ricci R. "Jnking" atherosclerosis. Cell Mol Life Sci 2005;62(21): 2487–94.

[98] Hirosumi J, Tuncman G, Chang L, et al. A central role for JNK in obesity and insulin resistance. Nature 2002;420(6913):333–6.

[99] Hotamisligil GS. Inflammatory pathways and insulin action. Int J Obes Relat Metab Disord 2003;27(Suppl 3):S53–5.

[100] Zelivianski S, Spellman M, Kellerman M, et al. ERK inhibitor PD98059 enhances docetaxel-induced apoptosis of androgen-independent human prostate cancer cells. Int J Cancer 2003;107(3):478–85.

[101] Ramesh G, Reeves WB. p38 MAP kinase inhibition ameliorates cisplatin nephrotoxicity in mice. Am J Physiol Renal Physiol 2005;289(1):F166–74.

[102] Yang SA, Paek SH, Kozukue N, et al. alpha-Chaconine, a potato glycoalkaloid, induces apoptosis of HT-29 human colon cancer cells through caspase-3 activation and inhibition of ERK 1/2 phosphorylation. Food Chem Toxicol 2006;44(6):839–46.

[103] Lamy S, Ruiz MT, Wisniewski J, et al. A prostate secretory protein94-derived synthetic peptide PCK3145 inhibits VEGF signalling in endothelial cells: implication in tumor angiogenesis. Int J Cancer 2006;118(9):2350–8.

[104] Waetzig V, Herdegen T. Context-specific inhibition of JNKs: overcoming the dilemma of protection and damage. Trends Pharmacol Sci 2005;26(9):455–61.

[105] Curtis TM, Scholfield CN. The role of lipids and protein kinase Cs in the pathogenesis of diabetic retinopathy. Diabetes Metab Res Rev 2004;20(1):28–43.

[106] Mochly-Rosen D, Khaner H, Lopez J. Identification of intracellular receptor proteins for activated protein kinase C. Proc Natl Acad Sci U S A 1991;88(9):3997–4000.

[107] Ginsberg HN, Illingworth DR. Postprandial dyslipidemia: an atherogenic disorder common in patients with diabetes mellitus. Am J Cardiol 2001;88(6A):9H–15H.

[108] Lebovitz HE. Effect of the postprandial state on nontraditional risk factors. Am J Cardiol 2001;88(6A):20H–5H.

[109] Ceriello A. Postprandial hyperglycemia and diabetes complications: is it time to treat? Diabetes 2005;54(1):1–7.

[110] Hoffman JM, Ishizuka T, Farese RV. Interrelated effects of insulin and glucose on diacylglycerol-protein kinase-C signalling in rat adipocytes and solei muscle in vitro and in vivo in diabetic rats. Endocrinology 1991;128(6):2937–48.

[111] Xia P, Inoguchi T, Kern TS, et al. Characterization of the mechanism for the chronic activation of diacylglycerol-protein kinase C pathway in diabetes and hypergalactosemia. Diabetes 1994;43(9):1122–9.

[112] Wautier MP, Chappey O, Corda S, et al. Activation of NADPH oxidase by AGE links oxidant stress to altered gene expression via RAGE. Am J Physiol Endocrinol Metab 2001;280(5):E685–94.

[113] Yan SD, Schmidt AM, Anderson GM, et al. Enhanced cellular oxidant stress by the interaction of advanced glycation end products with their receptors/binding proteins. J Biol Chem 1994;269(13):9889–97.

[114] Goldberg IJ. Lipoprotein lipase and lipolysis: central roles in lipoprotein metabolism and atherogenesis. J Lipid Res 1996;37(4):693–707.

[115] Morley NH, Kuksis A, Buchnea D, et al. Hydrolysis of diacylglycerols by lipoprotein lipase. J Biol Chem 1975;250(9):3414–8.

[116] Morley N, Kuksis A, Hoffman AG, et al. Preferential in vivo accumulation of sn-2, 3-diacylglycerols in postheparin plasma of rats. Can J Biochem 1977;55(10):1075–81.

[117] Lalanne F, Pruneta V, Bernard S, et al. Distribution of diacylglycerols among plasma lipoproteins in control subjects and in patients with non-insulin-dependent diabetes. Eur J Clin Invest 1999;29(2):139–44.

[118] Ishii H, Koya D, King GL. Protein kinase C activation and its role in the development of vascular complications in diabetes mellitus. J Mol Med 1998;76(1):21–31.

[119] Du X, Jiang Y, Qian W, et al. Fatty acids inhibit growth-factor-induced diacylglycerol kinase alpha activation in vascular smooth-muscle cells. Biochem J 2001;357(Pt 1):275–82.

[120] Khan WA, Blobe GC, Hannun YA. Arachidonic acid and free fatty acids as second messengers and the role of protein kinase C. Cell Signal 1995;7(3):171–84.

[121] McPhail LC, Clayton CC, Snyderman R. A potential second messenger role for unsaturated fatty acids: activation of Ca2+dependent protein kinase. Science 1984;224(4649): 622–5.

[122] el Touny S, Khan W, Hannun Y. Regulation of platelet protein kinase C by oleic acid. Kinetic analysis of allosteric regulation and effects on autophosphorylation, phorbol ester binding, and susceptibility to inhibition. J Biol Chem 1990;265(27):16437–43.

[123] Yaney GC, Korchak HM, Corkey BE. Long-chain acyl CoA regulation of protein kinase C and fatty acid potentiation of glucose-stimulated insulin secretion in clonal beta-cells. Endocrinology 2000;141(6):1989–98.

[124] Brawn MK, Chiou WJ, Leach KL. Oxidant-induced activation of protein kinase C in UC11MG cells. Free Radic Res 1995;22(1):23–37.

[125] Gopalakrishna R, Anderson WB. Ca2+ and phospholipid-independent activation of protein kinase C by selective oxidative modification of the regulatory domain. Proc Natl Acad Sci U S A 1989;86(17):6758–62.

[126] Palumbo EJ, Sweatt JD, Chen SJ, et al. Oxidation-induced persistent activation of protein kinase C in hippocampal homogenates. Biochem Biophys Res Commun 1992;187(3): 1439–45.

[127] Whisler RL, Goyette MA, Grants IS, et al. Sublethal levels of oxidant stress stimulate multiple serine/threonine kinases and suppress protein phosphatases in Jurkat T cells. Arch Biochem Biophys 1995;319(1):23–35.

[128] Gopalakrishna R, Anderson WB. Reversible oxidative activation and inactivation of protein kinase C by the mitogen/tumor promoter periodate. Arch Biochem Biophys 1991; 285(2):382–7.

[129] Gopalakrishna R, Jaken S. Protein kinase C signaling and oxidative stress. Free Radic Biol Med 2000;28(9):1349–61.

[130] Konishi H, Yamauchi E, Taniguchi H, et al. Phosphorylation sites of protein kinase C delta in H2O2-treated cells and its activation by tyrosine kinase in vitro. Proc Natl Acad Sci U S A 2001;98(12):6587–92.

[131] Yamamoto T, Matsuzaki H, Konishi H, et al. (2)O(2)-induced tyrosine phosphorylation of protein kinase cdelta by a mechanism independent of inhibition of protein-tyrosine phosphatase in CHO and COS-7 cells. Biochem Biophys Res Commun 2000;273(3):960–6.

[132] Way KJ, Katai N, King GL. Protein kinase C and the development of diabetic vascular complications. Diabet Med 2001;18(12):945–59.

[133] Ahmad FK, He Z, King GL. Molecular targets of diabetic cardiovascular complications. Curr Drug Targets 2005;6(4):487–94.

[134] Rask-Madsen C, King GL. Proatherosclerotic mechanisms involving protein kinase C in diabetes and insulin resistance. Arterioscler Thromb Vasc Biol 2005;25(3):487–96.

[135] Koya D, King GL. Protein kinase C activation and the development of diabetic complications. Diabetes 1998;47(6):859–66.

[136] King GL, Kunisaki M, Nishio Y, et al. Biochemical and molecular mechanisms in the development of diabetic vascular complications. Diabetes 1996;45(Suppl 3):S105–8.

[137] King GL, Brownlee M. The cellular and molecular mechanisms of diabetic complications. Endocrinol Metab Clin North Am 1996;25(2):255–70.

[138] Sheppard FR, Kelher MR, Moore EE, et al. Structural organization of the neutrophil NADPH oxidase: phosphorylation and translocation during priming and activation. J Leukoc Biol 2005;78(5):1025–42.

[139] Inoguchi T, Sonta T, Tsubouchi H, et al. Protein kinase C-dependent increase in reactive oxygen species (ROS) production in vascular tissues of diabetes: role of vascular NAD(P)H oxidase. J Am Soc Nephrol 2003;14(8, Suppl 3):S227–32.

[140] Inoguchi T, Nawata H. NAD(P)H oxidase activation: a potential target mechanism for diabetic vascular complications, progressive beta-cell dysfunction and metabolic syndrome. Curr Drug Targets 2005;6(4):495–501.

[141] Aronson D, Rayfield EJ. How hyperglycemia promotes atherosclerosis: molecular mechanisms. Cardiovasc Diabetol 2002;1:1.

[142] Brownlee M. The pathobiology of diabetic complications: a unifying mechanism. Diabetes 2005;54(6):1615–25.

[143] Nishikawa T, Edelstein D, Brownlee M. The missing link: a single unifying mechanism for diabetic complications. Kidney Int Suppl 2000;77:S26–30.

[144] Whiteside CI. Cellular mechanisms and treatment of diabetes vascular complications converge on reactive oxygen species. Curr Hypertens Rep 2005;7(2):148–54.

[145] Endemann DH, Schiffrin EL. Nitric oxide, oxidative excess, and vascular complications of diabetes mellitus. Curr Hypertens Rep 2004;6(2):85–9.

[146] Yagi N, Takasu N, Higa S, et al. Effect of troglitazone, a new oral antidiabetic agent, on fructose-induced insulin resistance. Horm Metab Res 1995;27:439–41.

[147] Ceriello A, Motz E. Is oxidative stress the pathogenic mechanism underlying insulin resistance, diabetes, and cardiovascular disease? The common soil hypothesis revisited. Arterioscler Thromb Vasc Biol 2004;24(5):816–23.

[148] Dandona P, Aljada A, Mohanty P, et al. Insulin inhibits intranuclear nuclear factor kappaB and stimulates IkappaB in mononuclear cells in obese subjects: evidence for an anti-inflammatory effect? J Clin Endocrinol Metab 2001;86(7):3257–65.

[149] Wolin MS, Ahmad M, Gupte SA. The sources of oxidative stress in the vessel wall. Kidney Int 2005;67(5):1659–61.

[150] Green K, Brand MD, Murphy MP. Prevention of mitochondrial oxidative damage as a therapeutic strategy in diabetes. Diabetes 2004;53(Suppl 1):S110–8.

[151] Weiss SJ, King GW, LoBuglio AF. Superoxide generation by human monocytes and macrophages. Am J Hematol 1978;4(1):1–8.

[152] Du X, Matsumura T, Edelstein D, et al. Inhibition of GAPDH activity by poly(ADP-ribose) polymerase activates three major pathways of hyperglycemic damage in endothelial cells. J Clin Invest 2003;112(7):1049–57.

[153] Robertson RP. Chronic oxidative stress as a central mechanism for glucose toxicity in pancreatic islet beta cells in diabetes. J Biol Chem 2004;279(41):42351–4.

[154] Lin KY, Ito A, Asagami T, et al. Impaired nitric oxide synthase pathway in diabetes mellitus: role of asymmetric dimethylarginine and dimethylarginine dimethylaminohydrolase. Circulation 2002;106(8):987–92.

[155] Seltzer HS. A summary of criticisms of the findings and conclusions of the University Group Diabetes Program (UGDP). Diabetes 1972;21(9):976–9.

[156] Abraira C, Colwell JA, Nuttall FQ, et al. Veterans Affairs Cooperative Study on glycemic control and complications in type II diabetes (VA CSDM). Results of the feasibility trial. Veterans Affairs Cooperative Study in Type II Diabetes. Diabetes Care 1995;18(8):1113–23.

[157] UK Prospective Diabetes Study (UKPDS) Group. Effect of intensive blood-glucose control with metformin on complications in overweight patients with type 2 diabetes (UKPDS 34). Lancet 1998;352(9131):854–65.

[158] Lo IC, Shih JM, Jiang MJ. Reactive oxygen species and ERK 1/2 mediate monocyte chemotactic protein-1-stimulated smooth muscle cell migration. J Biomed Sci 2005;12(2): 377–88.

[159] Napoli C, de Nigris F, Palinski W. Multiple role of reactive oxygen species in the arterial wall. J Cell Biochem 2001;82(4):674–82.

[160] Hundal RS, Petersen KF, Mayerson AB, et al. Mechanism by which high-dose aspirin improves glucose metabolism in type 2 diabetes. J Clin Invest 2002;109(10):1321–6.

[161] Smith SI. PPAR-gamma receptor agonists–a review of their role in diabetic management in Trinidad and Tobago. Mol Cell Biochem 2004;263(1–2):189–210.

[162] van Tits LJ, Arioglu-Oral E, Sweep CG, et al. Anti-inflammatory effects of troglitazone in nondiabetic obese subjects independent of changes in insulin sensitivity. Neth J Med 2005; 63(7):250–5.

[163] van Wijk JP, de Koning EJ, Castro Cabezas M, et al. Rosiglitazone improves postprandial triglyceride and free fatty acid metabolism in type 2 diabetes. Diabetes Care 2005;28(4): 844–9.

[164] Stephens NG, Parsons A, Schofield PM, et al. Randomised controlled trial of vitamin E in patients with coronary disease: Cambridge Heart Antioxidant Study (CHAOS). Lancet 1996;347(9004):781–6.

[165] Rapola JM, Virtamo J, Ripatti S, et al. Randomised trial of alpha-tocopherol and beta-carotene supplements on incidence of major coronary events in men with previous myocardial infarction. Lancet 1997;349(9067):1715–20.

[166] Christen WG, Gaziano JM, Hennekens CH. Design of Physicians' Health Study II–a randomized trial of beta-carotene, vitamins E and C, and multivitamins, in prevention of cancer, cardiovascular disease, and eye disease, and review of results of completed trials. Ann Epidemiol 2000;10(2):125–34.

[167] Lee IM, Cook NR, Gaziano JM, et al. Vitamin E in the primary prevention of cardiovascular disease and cancer: the Women's Health Study: a randomized controlled trial. JAMA 2005;294(1):56–65.

[168] Weiss RH, Fretland DJ, Baron DA, et al. Manganese-based superoxide dismutase mimetics inhibit neutrophil infiltration in vivo. J Biol Chem 1996;271(42):26149–56.

[169] Cuzzocrea S, Mazzon E, Dugo L, et al. Protective effects of a new stable, highly active SOD mimetic, M40401 in splanchnic artery occlusion and reperfusion. Br J Pharmacol 2001; 132(1):19–29.

[170] Salvemini D, Mazzon E, Dugo L, et al. Pharmacological manipulation of the inflammatory cascade by the superoxide dismutase mimetic, M40403. Br J Pharmacol 2001;132(4):815–27.

[171] Hink U, Li H, Mollnau H, et al. Mechanisms underlying endothelial dysfunction in diabetes mellitus. Circ Res 2001;88(2):E14–22.

[172] Lee ME, Dhadly MS, Temizer DH, et al. Regulation of endothelin-1 gene expression by Fos and Jun. J Biol Chem 1991;266(28):19034–9.

[173] Kouroedov A, Eto M, Joch H, et al. Selective inhibition of protein kinase Cbeta2 prevents acute effects of high glucose on vascular cell adhesion molecule-1 expression in human endothelial cells. Circulation 2004;110(1):91–6.

[174] Omi H, Okayama N, Shimizu M, et al. Participation of high glucose concentrations in neutrophil adhesion and surface expression of adhesion molecules on cultured human endothelial cells: effect of antidiabetic medicines. J Diabetes Complications 2002;16(3):201–8.

[175] Hall JL, Matter CM, Wang X, et al. Hyperglycemia inhibits vascular smooth muscle cell apoptosis through a protein kinase C-dependent pathway. Circ Res 2000;87(7):574–80.

[176] Cosentino F, Eto M, De Paolis P, et al. High glucose causes upregulation of cyclooxygenase-2 and alters prostanoid profile in human endothelial cells: role of protein kinase C and reactive oxygen species. Circulation 2003;107(7):1017–23.

ELSEVIER
SAUNDERS

Endocrinol Metab Clin N Am
35 (2006) 551–560

ENDOCRINOLOGY
AND METABOLISM
CLINICS
OF NORTH AMERICA

Endothelial Dysfunction and Its Role in Diabetic Vascular Disease

Martin M. Hartge, BPharm, Ulrich Kintscher, MD,
Thomas Unger, MD*

*Center for Cardiovascular Research, Institute for Pharmacology, Charité Berlin,
Hessische Strasse 3-4, 10115 Berlin, Germany*

The endothelium produces multiple mediators that not only regulate blood pressure, but also important physiological inflammatory processes such as the recruitment and activation of inflammatory cells. However, chronic exposure to certain stresses causes endothelial dysfunction, which is associated with impaired physiologic nitric oxide (NO) production and chronic inflammation. Low-density lipoprotein (LDL) cholesterol and oxidative stress play major roles in the impairment of endothelial function by reducing the bioavailability of NO and activating a proinflammatory state. Biomechanical forces on the endothelium, including low shear stress from disturbed blood flow and hypertension, also contribute to increased endothelium dysfunction. In the diabetic state additional mechanisms prominently exaggerate endothelial dysfunction. Insulin signaling is impaired in states of insulin resistance such as in type 2 diabetes, resulting in a marked decrease in NO bioavailability, and increased vascular inflammation, including enhanced expression of interleukin (IL) 6, vascular cell adhesion molecule 1 (VCAM-1), and monocyte chemoattractant protein 1 (MCP-1). Moreover, hyperglycaemia leads to increased formation of advanced glycation end products (AGE), which quench NO and impair endothelial function.

Endothelial function

The endothelium is the biggest organ of the body and builds the inner layer of blood vessels. In addition to its role as a mechanical lining, the

---

* Corresponding author.
E-mail address: thomas.unger@charite.de (T. Unger).

0889-8529/06/$ - see front matter © 2006 Elsevier Inc. All rights reserved.
doi:10.1016/j.ecl.2006.06.006
endo.theclinics.com

endothelium has many important biological functions. These include the regulation of leucocyte-adhesion, extravasation, and subendothelial accumulation; the prevention of platelet adhesion resulting in thrombotic processes; and the regulation of blood vessel patency for maintenance of appropriate blood flow. These functions are under tight hormonal control by numerous vasoactive substances. Mechanical stimuli such as shear stress and pressure complete this regulatory network. The response of the endothelium to these stimuli results in the release of agents that influence vasomotor function through endothelium-mediated relaxation of vascular smooth muscle; inhibition of platelet-aggregation; and the promotion of fibrinolysis, resulting in the dissolution of possible micro-thrombi to maintain normal blood flow.

As described above, one of the major functions of the endothelium is to ensure adequate blood flow. This process is regulated by the secretion of diverse substances, among which prostacyclin I_2 (PGI_2) and NO are the two main vasodilatators; others include endothelium-derived hyperpolarizing factor and C-type natriuretic peptide [1–3]. In addition to their vasomotor-regulatory function, PGI_2 and NO exert anti-aggregatory effects in platelets [4,5]. To counterbalance vasodilation during maintenance of regular blood flow, antagonists of vasodilatation named vasoconstrictors are secreted by the endothelium, including endothelin-1 (ET-1), angiotensin II (Ang II), thromboxane A_2, and reactive oxygen species (ROS) [6,7]. The normal maintenance of vascular patency and perfusion is mediated by the endothelium by release of NO and PGI_2. These agents increase the activities of guanylate- and adenylate-cyclase, respectively, increasing c-GMP and c-AMP levels, which inhibit platelet aggregation and thrombosis [3,8]. In addition, inhibition of thrombosis is mediated by endothelial expression and presentation of the cell surface protein thrombomodulin. Thrombomodulin binds thrombin, causing a configurational change that inhibits the conversion of fibrinogen into fibrin [9] and permits the activation of, protein C by thrombin, followed by inactivation of factor Va and VIIIa [10].

The endothelium also facilitates fibrinolysis to ensure vascular patency and perfusion. Active plasmin is formed after the secretion of tissue plasminogen activator (tPA) by the endothelium leading to fibrin degradation. In contrast, plasminogen activator inhibitor 1 (PAI 1), secreted by the endothelium and other tissues, inhibits tPA and functions as an antifibrinolytic agent.

All the functions listed above are tightly balanced during regular endothelial function, whereas major imbalances in these processes occur during endothelial dysfunction.

Endothelial dysfunction

Normal endothelial function is characterized by the maintenance of balanced vascular pressure, patency, and perfusion; inhibition of thrombosis;

and induction of fibrinolysis; whereas endothelial dysfunction is characterized by interactions of numerous proinflammatory processes; reduced vasodilation; and prothrombic properties. Multiple disease conditions are
initiated or associated with endothelial dysfunction, including hypertension,
coronary artery disease [11], congestive heart failure [12], and chronic renal
failure [13]. Endothelial dysfunction is also correlated with types 1 and 2 diabetes [14–18], likewise in normotensive, normoglycemic, first-degree relatives of patients with type 2 diabetes [19]. Finally, endothelial dysfunction
has been shown to correlate with the metabolic syndrome, dyslipidemia
[20], insulin resistance [21], obesity [22], hyperhomocysteinemia [23], sedentary lifestyle [24], and smoking [25]. These observations suggest that the
pathophysiology of endothelial dysfunction is complex and involves multiple
mechanisms.

The inflammatory state in association with type 2 diabetes, obesity, and endothelial dysfunction

Inflammatory conditions are frequently associated with type 2 diabetes
and obesity [26]. First described in 1993 by Hotamisligil and colleagues
[27], the concept of inflammation in relation to obesity and insulin resistance
was initiated by the observation that adipocyte expression of the proinflammatory cytokine tumor necrosis factor alpha (TNFα) was markedly increased in obese mice, and that neutralisation of TNFα led to an
improvement of insulin resistance. Other studies have shown a significant
correlation between body mass index (BMI) and plasma TNFα levels in
obese patients [28]. Additional work in the area of obesity has confirmed
that obesity is a state of chronic inflammation as indicated by increased
plasma concentrations of C-reactive protein (CRP) [29], (IL 6) [30], and
plasminogen activator inhibitor-1 (PAI 1) [31]. Recently, two adipocyte-spe-
cific proteins, adiponectin and leptin, have been shown to play major roles
in inflammatory conditions. Plasma adiponectin concentrations have an in-
verse relationship with adiposity, insulin resistance, diastolic pressure, triglyceride concentration, and TNFα receptor concentrations [32]. Leptin,
conversely, is elevated in obese humans, has proaggregatory effects on platelets, and may also regulate immune function by stimulation of inflammatory
responses in immune cells. Leptin has also been shown to induce oxidative
stress and inflammation in endothelial cells [33] and may induce hypertension through centrally mediated mechanisms [34–36].

The genesis of inflammation in obesity and type 2 diabetes may link inflammation and endothelial dysfunction. TNFα has been shown to inhibit
autophosphorylation of the insulin receptor (IR) on tyrosine residues, and
to induce serine-phosphorylation of insulin receptor substrate-1 (IRS-1),
which in turn causes adipocyte IR serine-phosphorylation and inhibits IR
tyrosine phosphorylation [37]. These processes and TNFα-mediated

down-regulation of the IR occur in endothelial cells, and contribute to impairment of the normal insulin response to simulate NO synthesis, resulting in endothelial dysfunction. One possible explanation for the close link between obesity, type 2 diabetes, inflammation, and endothelial dysfunction is the enhancement of inflammation by a diminished endothelial insulin response itself. Insulin exerts anti-inflammatory effects at the cellular and molecular levels in vitro and in vivo. Low-dose infusion of insulin has been shown to reduce reactive oxygen species (ROS) generation, to suppress NADPH oxidase expression and plasma Intercellular Adhesion Molecule-1 (ICAM-1) and MCP-1 concentrations. However, long-term insulin infusion (4 hours) in healthy subjects was associated with an induction of endothelial dysfunction.

The role of nitric oxide in the pathophysiology of endothelial dysfunction

Endothelial NO is one of the most important substances for the normal function of blood vessels. It promotes vasodilation, inhibits abnormal growth and inflammation, and exerts antiaggregatory effects on platelets. Reduced endothelium-derived NO expression has often been reported in the presence of impaired endothelial function. This may be caused by reduced activity of endothelial NO synthase (eNOS) as a result of increased levels of endogenous or exogenous inhibitors or a reduced availability of the substrate, L-arginine. NO is quenched by ROS to form peroxynitrite [38], which is a cytotoxic oxidant, and affects protein function, causing endothelial dysfunction through nitration of proteins. Peroxynitrite is an important mediator of LDL oxidation, emphasizing its proatherogenic role [39]. Moreover, peroxynitrite leads to degradation of the eNOS cofactor tetrahydrobiopterin (BH_4) [40], resulting in an "uncoupling" of eNOS activity. In diabetic mice, endothelial and cardiac dysfunction can be prevented by treatment with FP15, a novel peroxynitrite decomposition catalyst [41]. Oxidant excess also results in reduction of BH_4 to 7,8-dihydrobiopterin. When this occurs, formation of the active dimer of eNOS with oxygenase activity is decreased and production of NO is curtailed. Under these conditions, the reductase function of eNOS is activated to produce more ROS, so that eNOS shifts from an oxygenase-producing NO to a reductase-producing ROS, with the consequent exaggeration of oxidant excess and its deleterious effects on endothelial and vascular function [42]. Both in animal models of hypertension and hypertensive patients, oxidative excess seems to be associated with endothelial dysfunction, which is affirmed by monitoring of impaired endothelium-dependent vasodilation after use of antioxidants [43]. Human studies investigating effects of antioxidants like vitamins C and E in hypertensive populations have shown mostly significant antihypertensive effects. Clinical studies reported blood pressure–reducing actions of vitamin C [44,45]. In contrast, clinical data received from the Heart

Outcomes Prevention Evaluation (HOPE) trial [46] and the Collaborative Group of the Primary Prevention Project [47], in which hypertensive patients were treated with vitamin E (400 IU/d), did not demonstrate any clinically relevant effects on blood pressure. Reasons for these conflicting data may relate to the fact that in experimental studies, vitamin E is supplemented at higher doses (800 to 1000 IU/d) than those used in clinical trials (300 to 500 IU/d).

The influence of diabetes on endothelial dysfunction

The incidence of diabetes, particularly type 2 diabetes, is increasing at a rapid rate in industrialized westernized countries [48–51], and the increased prevalence of diabetes is closely related to aging and obesity. Diabetes is also closely linked to oxidative excess, resulting in diabetic endothelial dysfunction [52,53], although additional mechanisms may also trigger diabetic endothelial dysfunction. In states of insulin resistance, insulin signaling is altered, differently affecting the two major pathways emerging from the insulin receptor. The "phosphoinositide 3-kinase/Akt/protein kinase B" signaling pathway is prominently altered, resulting in a marked decrease of eNOS activation. In contrast, the "mitogen-activated protein kinase" pathway leading to mitogenic effects and growth is unaffected [54–57].

Hyperglycaemia promotes the formation of advanced glycation end-products (AGEs), which induce ROS and promote vascular inflammation by stimulating endothelial expression of IL 6, VCAM-1, and MCP-1 [58]. Acute hyperglycemia can reduce NO availability [59] and attenuate endothelium-dependent vasodilation in humans in vivo [60]. AGEs play an important role in these processes, since inhibition of AGE formation with aminoguanidine prevents NO depletion and sustains endothelial function [61].

Pathophysiology of cardiovascular disease in diabetes and its link to endothelial dysfunction

Cardiovascular disease (CVD), and in particular macrovascular disease, is the major cause of mortality and morbidity in patients with type 2 diabetes mellitus. In addition to dyslipidemia, hyperglycemia, hypercoagulation, hyperinsulinemia [62], and hypertension are present approximately twice as frequently in people with diabetes mellitus as in nondiabetic individuals.

Type 2 diabetes and the metabolic syndrome are characterized by several hemodynamic and metabolic abnormalities. Endothelial dysfunction plays a central role in these abnormalities and is evident before the onset of diabetes. Furthermore, dysfunction of the vascular endothelium plays an important role in the increased CVD risk found in persons with diabetes and hypertension [49,63]. The combination of diabetes and hypertension appears to correlate with decreased coronary flow responses compared with diabetes alone [64]. Diabetes-associated alterations in the vascular endothelium contributing to endothelial dysfunction include impairment of NO release, reduced NO responsiveness, elevated expression and plasma levels of vasoconstrictors such as angiotensin II and endothelin-1, increased adhesion molecule expression, and associated enhanced adhesion of platelets and monocytes to vascular endothelium. Endothelial expression of adhesion molecules is augmented by exposure to dyslipidemia, hypertensive plasma vasoconstrictor concentrations, and elevated adipose-derived proinflammatory cytokine levels, to promote leukocyte adhesion and vascular extravasation. Endothelial dysfunction occurs as the initiating step in atherogenesis and, as discussed above, the diabetes-associated augmentation of processes that lead to endothelial dysfunction explains at least part of the enhanced progression of CVD in type 2 diabetes.

Effects of thiazolidinedione treatment on endothelial dysfunction and cardiovascular disease

Thiazolidinediones (TZDs), so-called glitazones, function as insulin sensitizers through the peroxisome proliferator-activated receptor γ (PPARγ). They enhance the effects of insulin in metabolic target tissues (eg, in skeletal muscle, liver, and fat) and directly improve peripheral insulin resistance. PPARγ plays a regulatory role in the expression of genes involved in carbohydrate and lipid metabolism, and also effects adipocyte differentiation. PPARγ is expressed in all major cell types found in vascular lesions: endothelial cells, monocytes/macrophages, and vascular smooth muscle cells. Because TZDs reduce insulin resistance, it was logical to study the effects of TZDs to improve endothelial dysfunction. PPARγ activators directly improve endothelial function in diabetic patients, thereby blocking one of the earliest steps in atherogenesis [65]. Beneficial effects of glitazones on endothelial function could be mediated in a number of ways, including molecular effects related to PPARγ agonist actions, such as improvement of glycemic control and lowering circulating free-fatty acids, and via important anti-inflammatory effects on endothelial cells and leukocytes (Fig. 1).

In multiple studies, PPARγ ligands have also shown beneficial antiatherogenic effects [66], such as potent inhibition of inflammation, blockade of macrophage differentiation [67] and cytokine secretion, as well as inhibition of vascular smooth muscle-proliferation and migration. In addition, glitazone therapy improves a number of surrogate risk factors for atherosclerosis such as intima-media thickness and plasma cytokine and C-reactive protein levels. Recently, pioglitazone has been shown to reduce total mortality, stroke, and non-fatal myocardial infarction in high-risk diabetic patients proving the effectiveness of such a treatment [68].

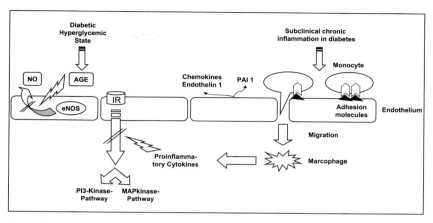

Fig. 1. Mechanisms involved in diabetic endothelial dysfunction. AGE, advanced glycation end products; eNOS, endothelial NO synthase; IR, insulin receptor; NO, nitric oxide; PAI 1, plasminogen activator inhibitor 1; TNF α, tumor necrosis factor α.

Summary

When the normal endothelial function is shifted in a pathological degree, the foundation is laid for possibly following diseases. This endothelial dysfunction is characterized by a proinflammatory state, reduced vasodilation, and a prothrombotic state. In the continuation, this dysfunction is strongly associated cardiovascular morbidity and mortality. Endothelial dysfunction is markedly enhanced in type 2 diabetes providing a major pathophysiological cause for the massively increased cardiovascular risk of diabetic patients. Subsequently future therapeutic approaches for the treatment of diabetic cardiovascular disease should target the dysfunctional endothelium first.

References

[1] Furchgott RF, Zawadzki JV. The obligatory role of endothelial cells in the relaxation of arterial smooth muscle by acetylcholine. Nature 1980;288(5789):373–6.
[2] Rovati GE, Giovanazzi S, Negretti A, et al. Prostacyclin effects on adenylate cyclase in platelets and vascular smooth muscle: interaction with an inhibitory receptor or partial agonism? Adv Prostaglandin Thromboxane Leukot Res 1995;23:263–5.
[3] Nicosia S, Oliva D, Bernini F, et al. Prostacyclin-sensitive adenylate cyclase and prostacyclin binding sites in platelets and smooth muscle cells. Adv Cyclic Nucleotide Protein Phosphorylation Res 1984;17:593–9.
[4] Grodzinska L, Marcinkiewicz E. The generation of TXA2 in human platelet rich plasma and its inhibition by nictindole and prostacyclin. Pharmacol Res Commun 1979;11(2):133–46.
[5] Barrett ML, Willis AL, Vane JR. Inhibition of platelet-derived mitogen release by nitric oxide (EDRF). Agents Actions 1989;27(3–4):488–91.

[6] Verma S, Anderson TJ. Fundamentals of endothelial function for the clinical cardiologist. Circulation 2002;105(5):546–9.

[7] Schiffrin EL. A critical review of the role of endothelial factors in the pathogenesis of hypertension. J Cardiovasc Pharmacol 2001;38(Suppl 2):S3–6.

[8] Riddell DR, Owen JS. Nitric oxide and platelet aggregation. Vitam Horm 1999;57:25–48.

[9] Wu KK, Thiagarajan P. Role of endothelium in thrombosis and hemostasis. Annu Rev Med 1996;47:315–31.

[10] van' Veer C, Golden NJ, Mann KG. Inhibition of thrombin generation by the zymogen factor VII: implications for the treatment of hemophilia A by factor VIIa. Blood 2000; 95(4):1330–5.

[11] Monnink SH, van Haelst PL, van Boven AJ, et al. Endothelial dysfunction in patients with coronary artery disease: a comparison of three frequently reported tests. J Investig Med 2002;50(1):19–24.

[12] Landmesser U, Spiekermann S, Dikalov S, et al. Vascular oxidative stress and endothelial dysfunction in patients with chronic heart failure: role of xanthine-oxidase and extracellular superoxide dismutase. Circulation 2002;106(24):3073–8.

[13] Bolton CH, Downs LG, Victory JG, et al. Endothelial dysfunction in chronic renal failure: roles of lipoprotein oxidation and pro-inflammatory cytokines. Nephrol Dial Transplant 2001;16(6):1189–97.

[14] Beckman JA, Goldfine AB, Gordon MB, et al. Oral antioxidant therapy improves endothelial function in Type 1 but not Type 2 diabetes mellitus. Am J Physiol Heart Circ Physiol 2003;285(6):H2392–8.

[15] Rizzoni D, Porteri E, Guelfi D, et al. Structural alterations in subcutaneous small arteries of normotensive and hypertensive patients with non-insulin-dependent diabetes mellitus. Circulation 2001;103(9):1238–44.

[16] Schofield I, Malik R, Izzard A, et al. Vascular structural and functional changes in type 2 diabetes mellitus: evidence for the roles of abnormal myogenic responsiveness and dyslipidemia. Circulation 2002;106(24):3037–43.

[17] Endemann DH, Pu Q, De Ciuceis C, et al. Persistent remodeling of resistance arteries in type 2 diabetic patients on antihypertensive treatment. Hypertension 2004;43(2):399–404.

[18] Panza JA, Quyyumi AA, Brush JE Jr, et al. Abnormal endothelium-dependent vascular relaxation in patients with essential hypertension. N Engl J Med 1990;323(1):22–7.

[19] Balletshofer BM, Rittig K, Enderle MD, et al. Endothelial dysfunction is detectable in young normotensive first-degree relatives of subjects with type 2 diabetes in association with insulin resistance. Circulation 2000;101(15):1780–4.

[20] Engler MM, Engler MB, Malloy MJ, et al. Antioxidant vitamins C and E improve endothelial function in children with hyperlipidemia: Endothelial Assessment of Risk from Lipids in Youth (EARLY) Trial. Circulation 2003;108(9):1059–63.

[21] Kim JA, Montagnani M, Koh KK, et al. Reciprocal relationships between insulin resistance and endothelial dysfunction: molecular and pathophysiological mechanisms. Circulation 2006;113(15):1888–904.

[22] Raitakari M, Ilvonen T, Ahotupa M, et al. Weight reduction with very-low-caloric diet and endothelial function in overweight adults: role of plasma glucose. Arterioscler Thromb Vasc Biol 2004;24(1):124–8.

[23] Virdis A, Ghiadoni L, Cardinal H, et al. Mechanisms responsible for endothelial dysfunction induced by fasting hyperhomocystinemia in normotensive subjects and patients with essential hypertension. J Am Coll Cardiol 2001;38(4):1106–15.

[24] Green DJ, Walsh JH, Maiorana A, et al. Exercise-induced improvement in endothelial dysfunction is not mediated by changes in CV risk factors: pooled analysis of diverse patient populations. Am J Physiol Heart Circ Physiol 2003;285(6):H2679–87.

[25] Oida K, Ebata K, Kanehara H, et al. Effect of cilostazol on impaired vasodilatory response of the brachial artery to ischemia in smokers. J Atheroscler Thromb 2003;10(2):93–8.

[26] Lehrke M, Lazar MA. Inflamed about obesity. Nat Med 2004;10(2):126–7.

[27] Hotamisligil GS, Shargill NS, Spiegelman BM. Adipose expression of tumor necrosis factor-alpha: direct role in obesity-linked insulin resistance. Science 1993;259(5091):87–91.

[28] Griendling KK, FitzGerald GA. Oxidative stress and cardiovascular injury: Part II: animal and human studies. Circulation 2003;108(17):2034–40.

[29] Yudkin JS, Stehouwer CD, Emeis JJ, et al. C-reactive protein in healthy subjects: associations with obesity, insulin resistance, and endothelial dysfunction: a potential role for cytokines originating from adipose tissue? Arterioscler Thromb Vasc Biol 1999;19(4):972–8.

[30] Mohamed-Ali V, Goodrick S, Rawesh A, et al. Subcutaneous adipose tissue releases interleukin-6, but not tumor necrosis factor-alpha, in vivo. J Clin Endocrinol Metab 1997;82(12): 4196–200.

[31] Lundgren CH, Brown SL, Nordt TK, et al. Elaboration of type-1 plasminogen activator inhibitor from adipocytes. A potential pathogenetic link between obesity and cardiovascular disease. Circulation 1996;93(1):106–10.

[32] Fernandez-Real JM, Lopez-Bermejo A, Casamitjana R, et al. Novel interactions of adiponectin with the endocrine system and inflammatory parameters. J Clin Endocrinol Metab 2003;88(6):2714–8.

[33] Matarese G, La Cava A, Sanna V, et al. Balancing susceptibility to infection and autoimmunity: a role for leptin? Trends Immunol 2002;23(4):182–7.

[34] Rahmouni K, Correia ML, Haynes WG, et al. Obesity-associated hypertension: new insights into mechanisms. Hypertension 2005;45(1):9–14.

[35] Hall JE, Hildebrandt DA, Kuo J. Obesity hypertension: role of leptin and sympathetic nervous system. Am J Hypertens 2001;14(6 Pt 2):103S–15S.

[36] Dunbar JC, Hu Y, Lu H. Intracerebroventricular leptin increases lumbar and renal sympathetic nerve activity and blood pressure in normal rats. Diabetes 1997;46(12):2040–3.

[37] Hotamisligil GS, Budavari A, Murray D, et al. Reduced tyrosine kinase activity of the insulin receptor in obesity-diabetes. Central role of tumor necrosis factor-alpha. J Clin Invest 1994; 94(4):1543–9.

[38] Koppenol WH, Moreno JJ, Pryor WA, et al. Peroxynitrite, a cloaked oxidant formed by nitric oxide and superoxide. Chem Res Toxicol 1992;5(6):834–42.

[39] Griendling KK, FitzGerald GA. Oxidative stress and cardiovascular injury: Part I: basic mechanisms and in vivo monitoring of ROS. Circulation 2003;108(16):1912–6.

[40] Milstien S, Katusic Z. Oxidation of tetrahydrobiopterin by peroxynitrite: implications for vascular endothelial function. Biochem Biophys Res Commun 1999;263(3):681–4.

[41] Szabo C, Mabley JG, Moeller SM, et al. Part I: pathogenetic role of peroxynitrite in the development of diabetes and diabetic vascular complications: studies with FP15, a novel potent peroxynitrite decomposition catalyst. Mol Med 2002;8(10):571–80.

[42] Landmesser U, Dikalov S, Price SR, et al. Oxidation of tetrahydrobiopterin leads to uncoupling of endothelial cell nitric oxide synthase in hypertension. J Clin Invest 2003;111(8): 1201–9.

[43] Chen X, Touyz RM, Park JB, et al. Antioxidant effects of vitamins C and E are associated with altered activation of vascular NADPH oxidase and superoxide dismutase in stroke-prone SHR. Hypertension 2001;38(3 Pt 2):606–11.

[44] Duffy SJ, Gokce N, Holbrook M, et al. Treatment of hypertension with ascorbic acid. Lancet 1999;354(9195):2048–9.

[45] Fotherby MD, Williams JC, Forster LA, et al. Effect of vitamin C on ambulatory blood pressure and plasma lipids in older persons. J Hypertens 2000;18(4):411–5.

[46] Hoogwerf BJ, Young JB. The HOPE study. Ramipril lowered cardiovascular risk, but vitamin E did not. Cleve Clin J Med 2000;67(4):287–93.

[47] Palumbo G, Avanzini F, Alli C, et al. Effects of vitamin E on clinic and ambulatory blood pressure in treated hypertensive patients. Collaborative Group of the Primary Prevention Project (PPP)–Hypertension study. Am J Hypertens 2000;13(5 Pt 1):564–7.

[48] Amos AF, McCarty DJ, Zimmet P. The rising global burden of diabetes and its complications: estimates and projections to the year 2010. Diabet Med 1997;14(Suppl 5):S1–85.

[49] Sowers JR. Diabetes mellitus and cardiovascular disease in women. Arch Intern Med 1998; 158(6):617–21.

[50] Muggeo M, Verlato G, Bonora E, et al. The Verona diabetes study: a population-based survey on known diabetes mellitus prevalence and 5-year all-cause mortality. Diabetologia 1995;38(3):318–25.

[51] Berger M, Jorgens V, Flatten G. Health care for persons with non-insulin-dependent diabetes mellitus. The German experience. Ann Intern Med 1996;124(1 Pt 2):153–5.

[52] Frisbee JC, Stepp DW. Impaired NO-dependent dilation of skeletal muscle arterioles in hypertensive diabetic obese Zucker rats. Am J Physiol Heart Circ Physiol 2001;281(3): H1304–11.

[53] Kim YK, Lee MS, Son SM, et al. Vascular NADH oxidase is involved in impaired endothelium-dependent vasodilation in OLETF rats, a model of type 2 diabetes. Diabetes 2002; 51(2):522–7.

[54] Cusi K, Maezono K, Osman A, et al. Insulin resistance differentially affects the PI 3-kinase- and MAP kinase-mediated signaling in human muscle. J Clin Invest 2000;105(3):311–20.

[55] Montagnani M, Ravichandran LV, Chen H, et al. Insulin receptor substrate-1 and phosphoinositide-dependent kinase-1 are required for insulin-stimulated production of nitric oxide in endothelial cells. Mol Endocrinol 2002;16(8):1931–42.

[56] Osman AA, Pendergrass M, Koval J, et al. Regulation of MAP kinase pathway activity in vivo in human skeletal muscle. Am J Physiol Endocrinol Metab 2000;278(6):E992–9.

[57] Federici M, Menghini R, Mauriello A, et al. Insulin-dependent activation of endothelial nitric oxide synthase is impaired by O-linked glycosylation modification of signaling proteins in human coronary endothelial cells. Circulation 2002;106(4):466–72.

[58] Zhang L, Zalewski A, Liu Y, et al. Diabetes-induced oxidative stress and low-grade inflammation in porcine coronary arteries. Circulation 2003;108(4):472–8.

[59] Giugliano D, Marfella R, Coppola L, et al. Vascular effects of acute hyperglycemia in humans are reversed by L-arginine. Evidence for reduced availability of nitric oxide during hyperglycemia. Circulation 1997;95(7):1783–90.

[60] Williams SB, Goldfine AB, Timimi FK, et al. Acute hyperglycemia attenuates endothelium-dependent vasodilation in humans in vivo. Circulation 1998;97(17):1695–701.

[61] Bucala R, Tracey KJ, Cerami A. Advanced glycosylation products quench nitric oxide and mediate defective endothelium-dependent vasodilatation in experimental diabetes. J Clin Invest 1991;87(2):432–8.

[62] Sowers JR. Hypertension in Type II diabetes: update on therapy. J Clin Hypertens (Greenwich) 1999;1(1):41–7.

[63] Sowers JR, Epstein M. Diabetes mellitus and associated hypertension, vascular disease, and nephropathy. An update. Hypertension 1995;26(6 Pt 1):869–79.

[64] Prior JO, Quinones MJ, Hernandez-Pampaloni M, et al. Coronary circulatory dysfunction in insulin resistance, impaired glucose tolerance, and type 2 diabetes mellitus. Circulation 2005;111(18):2291–8.

[65] Hsueh WA, Lyon CJ, Quinones MJ. Insulin resistance and the endothelium. Am J Med 2004; 117(2):109–17.

[66] Collins A, Noh G. PPARgamma ligands attenuate angiotensin-II accelerated atherosclerosis in male low density receptor deficient (LDLR/) mice. Diabetes 2001;50.

[67] Ricote M, Li AC, Willson TM, et al. The peroxisome proliferator-activated receptor-gamma is a negative regulator of macrophage activation. Nature 1998;391(6662):79–82.

[68] Dormandy JA, Charbonnel B, Eckland DJ, et al. Secondary prevention of macrovascular events in patients with type 2 diabetes in the PROactive Study (PROspective pioglitAzone Clinical Trial In macroVascular Events): a randomised controlled trial. Lancet 2005; 366(9493):1279–89.

ELSEVIER
SAUNDERS

Endocrinol Metab Clin N Am
35 (2006) 561–574

ENDOCRINOLOGY
AND METABOLISM
CLINICS
OF NORTH AMERICA

Peroxisome Proliferator-Activated Receptor Gamma Agonists: Their Role as Vasoprotective Agents in Diabetes

Florian Blaschke, MD, Evren Caglayan, MD,
Willa A. Hsueh, MD*

*Department of Endocrinology, Diabetes and Metabolism, Division of Endocrinology,
Diabetes and Hypertension, David Geffen School of Medicine,
University of California, 900 Veteran Avenue, Warren Hall, Suite 24-130,
Los Angeles, CA 90095, USA*

The incidence of type 2 diabetes is increasing dramatically in Western industrialized societies because of increasing obesity, sedentary lifestyle, and an aging population. Diabetes mellitus is associated with an increased risk of developing atherosclerotic vascular disorders (including coronary, cerebrovascular, and peripheral artery disease) and cardiovascular disease accounts for up to 80% of premature excess mortality in diabetic patients [1]. Consequently, both type 1 and type 2 diabetes are considered a coronary artery disease (CAD) risk equivalent [2]. Metabolic syndrome, a constellation of metabolic alterations associated with obesity, sedentary lifestyle, and ethnic background, is a major risk factor for subsequent development of type 2 diabetes and CAD, and is defined by the National Cholesterol Education Program Adult Treatment Panel III [2] as three or more of the following five conditions:

- Fasting hyperglycemia (≥ 110 mg/dl)
- Hypertension ($\geq 130/85$ mm Hg)
- Hypertriglyceridemia (≥ 150 mg/dl)
- Reduced high-density lipoprotein (HDL; men < 40/mg/dl; women < 50 mg/dl)
- Increased waist circumference (men > 102 cm; women > 88 cm)

Insulin resistance, defined as a defect in the ability of insulin to drive glucose into its major target tissue, skeletal muscle [3], is usually a component

* Corresponding author.
E-mail address: whsueh@mednet.ucla.edu (W.A. Hsueh).

of the metabolic syndrome. It is a key factor in the pathogenesis of type 2 diabetes and a cofactor in the development of dyslipidemia, hypertension, and atherosclerosis [4]. Insulin resistance is present in more than 90% of people with type 2 diabetes and predates the development of hyperglycemia by many years [5]. Other components of the metabolic syndrome (ie, hypertension, hypertriglyceridemia, and decreased HDL) are themselves CAD risk factors, and hyperglycemia further contributes to vascular damage. Whether or not hyperinsulinemia and insulin resistance directly contribute to vascular damage is controversial and under active investigation [6].

The pathogenesis of CAD in diabetes is multifactorial. Metabolic changes, oxidative stress and glycoxidation, endothelial dysfunction, inflammation, and a diabetes-associated prothrombotic state all play a role in the cardiovascular complications of diabetes [7]. For example, current evidence suggests a pivotal role for inflammation in all phases of atherosclerosis, from the formation of fatty streaks to subsequent rupture of the lesions and acute coronary syndromes [8,9]. This concept is supported by epidemiologic and clinical studies, where systemic inflammatory markers, such as C-reactive protein (CRP), interleukin-6 (IL-6), and serum amyloid A, have been shown to be strong predictors of cardiovascular complications in various settings [10]. In addition to the potential use of inflammatory biomarkers as risk predictors for cardiovascular events, they might serve as targets for pharmacologic therapy.

Diabetes mellitus is also associated with poor outcomes after vascular occlusion, compared with the nondiabetic population [11–13]. Plaque composition is known to determine the risk of plaque disruption and thrombosis, which is the main cause of acute coronary syndrome [14,15]. Plaques prone to rupture are characterized by decreased collagen and vascular smooth muscle cells (VSMCs) in their cap and shoulder regions, and a rich inflammatory infiltrate [16–18]. Atherosclerotic lesions of type 2 diabetic patients reveal greater macrophage infiltration, larger lipid cores, and decreased VSMC content than lesions from nondiabetic patients [19]. Thus, type 2 diabetes is associated not only with accelerated and premature coronary atherosclerosis, but also with an increased vulnerability for plaque rupture and thrombosis [20]. The United Kingdom Prospective Diabetes Study [21] demonstrated that intensive blood glucose control with insulin or sulfonylurea in type 2 diabetic subjects had only a limited effect on the incidence of cardiovascular events, indicating the necessity of new treatment strategies to reduce cardiovascular morbidity and mortality associated with this syndrome.

Thiazolidinediones and peroxisome proliferator-activated receptors

Thiazolidinediones (TZDs), a class of insulin-sensitizing agents that act as ligands for the nuclear receptor peroxisome proliferator-activated receptor gamma (PPAR-γ), are used frequently in the treatment of patients who have type 2 diabetes. These drugs reduce peripheral insulin resistance, characteristically found in type 2 diabetic patients, by increasing insulin-dependent glucose disposal and reducing hepatic glucose output [22]. The first clinically used TZD, Troglitazone, was withdrawn from the market because of rare, but serious hepatotoxicity [23]. Rosiglitazone and pioglitazone, the two TZDs currently available, are not associated with any hepatotoxicity and are used widely for treatment of type 2 diabetes [24]. In addition to their effects on carbohydrate metabolism, TZDs have beneficial effects on plasma lipids. Both pioglitazone and rosiglitazone increase serum levels of HDL [25,26], and pioglitazone also markedly reduces plasma triglyceride levels [27]. In addition, in numerous studies, TZDs and non-TZD PPAR-γ ligands have been found to attenuate atherosclerotic lesion formation in animal models and reduce inflammatory gene expression in vascular cells in vitro [28–31].

PPARs, which are ligand-activated transcription factors belonging to the nuclear receptor superfamily, regulate the transcription of target genes by forming heterodimers with the retinoid X receptor (RXR) and binding to specific PPAR response elements in the promoter region of target genes [32,33]. Three isoforms, PPAR-γ, PPAR-α, and PPAR-δ, which share 60% to 80% homology in their ligand- and DNA-binding domains, have been identified so far. Unsaturated long-chain fatty acids and their eicosanoids derivatives are endogenous ligands for all three PPAR isotypes [34,35]. Synthetic ligands for two of these, PPAR-α and PPAR-γ, have been developed for clinical use; ligands for PPAR-δ are currently under clinical development. In the absence of ligands, PPAR/RXR heterodimers have the potential to actively repress transcription through the recruitment of corepressor complexes containing the nuclear receptor corepressor (NCoR) or the silencing mediator of retinoid and thyroid receptors (SMRT) [36,37]. Ligand binding induces a conformational change in the heterodimeric unit, which activates gene transcription through dissociation of corepressors and recruitment of coactivators [38]. PPARs can also repress gene expression in a DNA-binding–independent manner, by antagonizing the activities of other signal-dependent transcription factors such as nuclear factor–kappaB (NF-κB) and activator protein-1 (AP-1) [39].

Role of peroxisome proliferator-activated receptor gamma in adipose tissue

Adipose tissue is an endocrine organ that releases proinflammatory factors that promote vascular damage and atherosclerosis. Tumor necrosis factor alpha (TNF-α) inhibits insulin signaling, thereby contributing to insulin resistance, and activates multiple proinflammatory pathways via NF-κB [40]. Leptin, produced by adipose tissue, can alter insulin action and has been recognized recently to be an important mediator of obesity-related hypertension [41]. In contrast, visceral adipose tissue increases are associated with decreased plasma adiponectin [42], a protein recently shown to have significant antidiabetic and anti-atherogenic functions [43,44]. Taken together, these observations indicate that the adipocyte plays a central role in the relationship between obesity, diabetes, and CAD.

PPAR-γ, the molecular target of the TZD ligands, is expressed at high levels in adipose tissue, and is a central regulator of adipocyte gene expression and differentiation [45,46]. Retroviral-mediated expression of PPAR-γ stimulates adipose differentiation of cultured fibroblasts [47], and several studies have demonstrated that PPAR-γ expression is necessary and sufficient to promote adipocyte cell differentiation in vivo and in vitro [48,49].

Although the mechanisms underlying the insulin-sensitizing effects of TZDs are complex and not understood completely, adipose tissue is known to be an important target of TZDs. Activation of PPAR-γ in insulin-resistant animals or humans results in an increase in the sensitivity of the liver to insulin-mediated suppression of hepatic glucose production and the skeletal muscle to insulin-mediated glucose uptake [50,51]. These in vivo effects on insulin signaling are caused by the combined actions of PPAR-γ ligands on adipose tissue, liver, and skeletal muscle. A significant role for adipose tissue in insulin sensitization was found initially in a study that revealed that the TZD rosiglitazone does not reduce glucose or insulin levels in insulin-resistant mice lacking white adipose tissue, suggesting that white adipose tissue is required for the antidiabetic effects of PPAR-γ ligands [52].

PPAR-γ ligands profoundly alter gene expression in adipose tissue. Resistin and TNF-α expression, both of which induce insulin resistance, are reduced by PPAR-γ ligands, suggesting that the insulin-sensitizing effects of PPAR-γ agonists are related to their anti-inflammatory properties [53,54]. In addition, expression and secretion of adiponectin, a protein produced exclusively by the adipocyte, is increased by PPAR-γ agonists both in vivo and in vitro [55]. Altering pro- and anti-inflammatory protein secretion from adipose tissue thus appears to be an important mechanism whereby TZDs improve insulin sensitivity in distant organs, and exert vasoprotective effects. These data suggest that adipose tissue may be the primary target of PPAR-γ ligands, resulting in improved insulin sensitivity in liver and muscle [56]. However, in recent studies, PPAR-γ ligands were found to improve insulin sensitivity in several different mouse models lacking adipose tissue, indicating a beneficial effect outside the adipose tissue [57,58]. Consistent with these observations, mice deficient in skeletal muscle or liver PPAR-γ expression have severe whole-body insulin resistance [59,60]. Hevener and colleagues [59] postulated that selective deletion of PPAR-γ in skeletal muscle caused insulin resistance in muscle, followed by impaired insulin action in adipose tissue and liver. In contrast, Norris and colleagues [61] found that in mice with muscle-specific deletion of PPAR-γ, insulin sensitivity in skeletal muscle was normal, but was impaired in the liver. Many of the differences in the mouse studies may depend on strain differences.

Role of peroxisome proliferator-activated receptor gamma in inflammation and atherosclerosis

In addition to adipose tissue, liver, and skeletal muscle, PPAR-γ is expressed in VSMCs, endothelial cells, macrophages, and T-cells, where it plays an important role in regulating inflammatory responses [30,39,62,63]. PPAR-γ–specific ligands inhibit the production of a host of inflammatory cytokines, such as TNF-α, IL-1-β and IL-6 in monocytes [30]; inducible nitric oxide synthase, matrix metalloproteinase 9, and scavenger receptor 1 in macrophages [39]; or endothelin-1 and interferon-inducible protein 10 (IP-10) in endothelial cells [64,65]. Moreover, PPAR-γ agonists have been shown to decrease the expression of the adhesive, proinflammatory molecule, osteopontin, in macrophages [66]. Previous studies suggest that the anti-inflammatory properties of PPAR-γ are caused by a generalized repression of NF-κB, CCAAT/enhancer binding protein (C/EBP), and AP-1 mediated gene transcription [67,68]. A recent report by Pascual and colleagues [31] suggests a novel mechanism, wherein ligand-dependent SUMOylation of the PPAR-γ ligand-binding domain targets PPAR-γ to nuclear receptor corepressor complexes on proinflammatory gene promoters, stabilizing these complexes to maintain transcriptional repression.

Studies examining the anti-inflammatory effects of PPAR-γ in mouse models of inflammation have yielded mixed results. For example, PPAR-γ ligands markedly reduced colonic inflammation in a mouse model of inflammatory bowel disease [69], and significantly reduced TNF-α and gelatinase B mRNA expression in the aortic root of mice [28]. However, PPAR-γ ligands did not attenuate lipopolysaccharide (LPS)-induced cytokine production significantly in a mouse inflammation model [28]. Moreover, some anti-inflammatory effects required high ligand doses and did not appear to be mediated by receptor-dependent processes [70].

In various studies, PPAR-γ ligands have been shown to decrease atherosclerotic lesion formation in genetically prone mouse models [28,29,71,72]. This effect occurs in insulin-sensitive and insulin-resistant models, with or without diabetes. Female mice demonstrate proportionally less attenuation of atherosclerosis upon PPAR-γ ligand treatment than male mice [28], indicating that additional factors such as hormonal status may affect the outcome. PPAR-γ ligands also inhibited angiotensin II (AngII)-accelerated atherosclerosis in low-density lipoprotein receptor knockout (LDLR$^{-/-}$) mice without effects on lipid profile, glucose, or blood pressure. The attenuation of AngII-accelerated atherosclerosis correlated with a downregulation of the proinflammatory transcription factor early growth response gene 1 (Egr-1) and several of its target genes [73], indicating that inhibition of inflammation plays a crucial role for the antiatherosclerotic effect of PPAR-γ ligands. AngII is known to be a major proatherogenic factor that induces inflammation in the vessel wall and stimulates proliferation and migration of VSMCs and monocytes [74–76]. Previous studies have shown that PPAR-γ ligands modulate AngII signaling both at the receptor level and downstream of the AngII type 1 receptor (AT(1)-R). PPAR-γ activators have been found to downregulate AT(1)-R expression in VSMCs and block AT(1)-R–mediated mitogen activated protein kinase ERK 1/2 activation, which is crucial for VSMC proliferation and migration [77,78]. However, various in vitro studies regarding the effect of PPAR-γ agonists on cholesterol homeostasis in macrophages suggest both atherogenic and antiatherogenic influences. PPAR-γ has been shown to transcriptionally induce the expression of the macrophage scavenger receptor CD36, suggesting that PPAR-γ might promote foam cell formation and the development of atherosclerosis [79,80]. However, Chawla and colleagues [81] demonstrated that, in addition to lipid uptake, PPAR-γ induces ATP binding cassette A-1 (ABCA1) expression and cholesterol efflux in macrophages through a transcriptional cascade mediated by liver X receptor alpha (LXR-α). Li and colleagues [82] recently demonstrated that PPAR-γ ligands inhibit the formation of macrophage foam cells in the peritoneal cavity of hypercholesterolemic LDLR$^{-/-}$ mice, possibly through transcriptional regulation of ABCG1, a transporter that mediates cholesterol efflux to HDL acceptors [83].

Results from the first TZD cardiovascular outcome trial, Prospective Pioglitazone Clinical Trial in Macrovascular Events (PROactive), were published recently [84]. In this prospective, double-blind, randomized, placebo-controlled, secondary prevention study, pioglitazone treatment was found to reduce the composite of all-cause mortality, nonfatal myocardial infarction, and stroke in type 2 diabetic subjects. Clinical trials examining shorter-term surrogate end points for atherosclerosis have revealed that TZD treatment improves measures of carotid intimal medial thickness [85,86]. TZDs may also improve endothelial reactivity. The authors' group recently demonstrated that rosiglitazone treatment improved positron emission tomography–assessed myocardial blood flow responses to cold pressor test, which is largely endothelial-dependent [87]. In addition, various studies have shown that treatment of subjects with type 2 diabetes with TZDs reduced inflammatory surrogate parameters of atherosclerosis, such as CRP, TNF-α serum amyloid A, and plasminogen activator inhibitor type-1 (PAI-1), while increasing adiponectin [54,55,88–90]. Although these effects where observed as early as 2 weeks after treatment, TZDs exhibit maximal glucose-lowering effects 8 to 12 weeks after start of treatment. Satoh and colleagues [89] observed that pioglitazone treatment reduced CRP levels in both responders and nonresponders with respect to its antidiabetic effect. These findings suggest that the effect of TZDs on the biomarkers of cardiovascular risk may be independent of their antidiabetic actions [91]. Previous data indicate that throughout the spectrum of insulin resistance, from the metabolic syndrome to type 2 diabetes, PAI-1 levels are increased [92]. Because PAI-1 promotes clot formation in plasma and various studies have demonstrated an association between circulating PAI-1 levels and cardiovascular events [93], a TZD-mediated decrease in PAI-1 might play an important role in reducing the incidence of CAD and its complications in this population.

Role of peroxisome proliferator-activated receptor gamma in restenosis

VSMC activation, migration, and proliferation not only play decisive roles in the development of atherosclerosis, but are also the primary pathophysiologic mechanism for the failure of procedures used to treat occlusive proliferative atherosclerotic diseases, such as postangioplasty restenosis, transplant vasculopathy, and vein bypass graft failure [94,95]. Patients who have diabetes are at increased risk not only for the development of CAD, but also have an elevated risk of developing postangioplasty restenosis, compared with individuals who do not have diabetes [13,96]. In response to vascular injury endothelial cells, VSMCs and macrophages secrete cytokines and growth factors that perpetuate the vasculoproliferative response.

PPAR-γ ligands have been shown to inhibit proliferation and migration of VSMCs in vivo [62,75]. The antiproliferative activity of PPAR-γ ligands appears to result from their ability to inhibit retinoblastoma protein (Rb) phosphorylation by modulating the expression of several key cell cycle regulators that control $G_1 \rightarrow S$ phase progression. Progression through the cell cycle requires cyclin/CDK complexes to phosphorylate Rb, which acts as a transition point for progression into S phase [97]. Phosphorylation of Rb in the late G_1 phase releases the S phase transcription factor E2F to induce the gene expression required for DNA synthesis and cell cycle progression [98]. Attenuation of mitogen-induced degradation of p27^{Kip1} by TZDs appears to be the major mechanism that ultimately leads to inhibition of Rb phosphorylation, E2F release, and E2F-dependent transactivation of gene expression. Migration of VSMCs into and within the intima requires the degradation of basal laminae and interstitial extracellular matrix by matrix metalloproteinase (MMP) activity, and PPAR-γ activation has been shown to inhibit expression and functional activity of MMP-9 [62], at least in part by attenuating the expression of the Ets-1 transcription factor [99].

Inhibition of VSMC growth and migration by PPAR-γ ligands in vitro turns into an in vivo alteration of neointima formation. In animal models of restenosis, TZDs have been shown to inhibit intimal hyperplasia after mechanical injury in both insulin-sensitive and insulin-resistant animals [100,101]. Moreover, early clinical trials of subjects with type 2 diabetes have demonstrated that both pioglitazone and rosiglitazone have a potent inhibitory effect on neointimal tissue formation after coronary stent implantation [102,103].

Summary

Obesity and diabetes mellitus, significant risk factors for the development of CAD, are becoming a global epidemic. Currently, CAD is the leading cause of death in the United States, accounting for approximately 500,000 deaths each year [104]. Despite significant improvements in the management of diabetes, type 2 diabetes mellitus remains a risk equivalent for CAD. A type 2 diabetic patient has the same risk of a future cardiovascular event as a nondiabetic individual who has had a prior myocardial infarction [20]. New treatment strategies are needed urgently to reduce diabetes-associated cardiovascular morbidity and mortality.

TZDs have demonstrated some cardiovascular benefits in early trials, and theoretically may improve cardiovascular disease risk through several mechanisms. PPAR-γ ligands have been shown to attenuate inflammatory responses, which have been shown to be associated with both insulin resistance and atherosclerosis. In addition, PPAR-γ agonists have been shown to induce ABCA1 and ABCG1 expression, potentially altering cholesterol efflux from macrophages. Inhibition of VSMC proliferation and migration, fundamental processes involved in atherosclerosis and restenosis, may contribute further to the potential cardiovascular benefit of these ligands.

Although current TZD PPAR-γ ligands may have significant potential benefits in the treatment of type 2 diabetes, these must be offset against potentially serious side effects. In clinical trials, both pioglitazone and rosiglitazone have been associated with fluid retention, hemodilution, weight gain, and congestive heart failure (CHF) [105]. The observed, normally modest weight gain is explained by fluid retention, increased adipogenesis, and a net flux of fatty acids into adipose tissue. However, these side effects were more apparent when TZDs were used in combination with insulin, and appeared to correlate with drug dosage. For example, rosiglitazone (4 or 8 mg/d) added to insulin therapy resulted in CHF rates of 2% and 3%, respectively, compared with a rate of 1% in the group treated with insulin alone [106,107]. Thus, according to American Heart Association and American Diabetes Association guidelines, TZDs should not be used in patients who have NYHA class III or IV CHF [108]. Another potential concern is the possibility that TZDs may promote tumorigenesis or tumor growth, because PPAR-γ ligands have been shown to increase the frequency and size of colon tumors in mice [109]. However, PPAR-γ agonists have also been shown to cause a significant reduction in the growth of human cancer cell lines [110]. Extrapolation of the evidence of carcinogenesis from rodents to humans is an uncertain process, and further studies are necessary.

The vascular effects of TZDs and their beneficial activity against multiple proinflammatory and prothrombotic factors provide a compelling rationale for conducting cardiovascular outcomes trials with these oral antidiabetic agents. In clinical studies, TZD treatment has been found to decrease carotid intimal medial wall thickness in type 2 diabetic subjects at 3- and 6-month end points [85,86]. In addition, clinical trials have shown that after coronary stent implantation, type 2 diabetics who received TZDs had a significant reduction in restenosis, compared with a control group who received equal glucose-lowering therapy with other agents [102,103]. Results from the first TZD cardiovascular outcome trial, PROactive, demonstrated that pioglitazone reduced the risk of all-cause mortality, myocardial infarction (excluding silent myocardial infarction), and stroke in subjects with type 2 diabetes. The cardiovascular outcomes trials RECORD (Rosiglitazone Evaluation for Cardiac Outcomes and Regulation of Glycemia in Diabetes) and BARI-2D (Bypass Angioplasty Revascularization Investigation in Type 2 Diabetes), using rosiglitazone, will help to determine whether the vascular and metabolic effects of PPAR-γ ligands can protect persons with type 2 diabetes from the increased atherothrombotic risk associated with that disease.

References

[1] Winer N, Sowers JR. Epidemiology of diabetes. J Clin Pharmacol 2004;44:397–405.
[2] Executive summary of the third report of The National Cholesterol Education Program (NCEP) Expert Panel on Detection, Evaluation, and Treatment of High Blood Cholesterol in Adults (Adult Treatment Panel III). JAMA 2001;285:2486–97.
[3] Saltiel AR, Kahn CR. Insulin signaling and the regulation of glucose and lipid metabolism. Nature 2001;414:799–806.
[4] Pi-Sunyer FX. The obesity epidemic: pathophysiology and consequences of obesity. Obes Res 2002;10(Suppl 2):97S–104S.
[5] Haffner SM, Stern MP, Hazuda HP, et al. Cardiovascular risk factors in confirmed prediabetic individuals. Does the clock for coronary heart disease start ticking before the onset of clinical diabetes? JAMA 1990;263:2893–8.
[6] Sjoholm A, Nystrom T. Endothelial inflammation in insulin resistance. Lancet 2005;365: 610–2.
[7] Eckel RH, Wassef M, Chait A, et al. Prevention Conference VI: Diabetes and Cardiovascular Disease: Writing Group II: pathogenesis of atherosclerosis in diabetes. Circulation 2002;105:e138–43.
[8] Ross R. Atherosclerosis–an inflammatory disease. N Engl J Med 1999;340:115–26.
[9] Libby P. Inflammation in atherosclerosis. Nature 2002;420:868–74.
[10] Ridker PM, Hennekens CH, Buring JE, et al. C-reactive protein and other markers of inflammation in the prediction of cardiovascular disease in women. N Engl J Med 2000;342: 836–43.
[11] Kannel WB, McGee DL. Diabetes and cardiovascular disease. The Framingham study. JAMA 1979;241:2035–8.
[12] Wei M, Gaskill SP, Haffner SM, et al. Effects of diabetes and level of glycemia on all-cause and cardiovascular mortality. The San Antonio heart study. Diabetes Care 1998;21: 1167–72.
[13] Kornowski R, Mintz GS, Kent KM, et al. Increased restenosis in diabetes mellitus after coronary interventions is due to exaggerated intimal hyperplasia. A serial intravascular ultrasound study. Circulation 1997;95:1366–9.
[14] Falk E, Shah PK, Fuster V. Coronary plaque disruption. Circulation 1995;92:657–71.
[15] Libby P. Molecular bases of the acute coronary syndromes. Circulation 1995;91:2844–50.
[16] Lendon CL, Davies MJ, Born GV, et al. Atherosclerotic plaque caps are locally weakened when macrophages density is increased. Atherosclerosis 1991;87:87–90.
[17] Moreno PR, Falk E, Palacios IF, et al. Macrophage infiltration in acute coronary syndromes. Implications for plaque rupture. Circulation 1994;90:775–8.
[18] van der Wal AC, Becker AE, van der Loos CM, et al. Site of intimal rupture or erosion of thrombosed coronary atherosclerotic plaques is characterized by an inflammatory process irrespective of the dominant plaque morphology. Circulation 1994;89:36–44.

[19] Moreno PR, Murcia AM, Palacios IF, et al. Coronary composition and macrophage infiltration in atherectomy specimens from patients with diabetes mellitus. Circulation 2000; 102:2180–4.

[20] Haffner SM, Lehto S, Ronnemaa T, et al. Mortality from coronary heart disease in subjects with type 2 diabetes and in nondiabetic subjects with and without prior myocardial infarction. N Engl J Med 1998;339:229–34.

[21] UK Prospective Diabetes Study (UKPDS) Group. Intensive blood-glucose control with sulphonylureas or insulin compared with conventional treatment and risk of complications in patients with type 2 diabetes (UKPDS 33). Lancet 1998;352:837–53.

[22] Saltiel AR, Olefsky JM. Thiazolidinediones in the treatment of insulin resistance and type II diabetes. Diabetes 1996;45:1661–9.

[23] Tolman KG, Chandramouli J. Hepatotoxicity of the thiazolidinediones. Clin Liver Dis 2003;7:369–79 [vi].

[24] Lehmann JM, Moore LB, Smith-Oliver TA, et al. An antidiabetic thiazolidinedione is a high affinity ligand for peroxisome proliferator-activated receptor gamma (PPAR gamma). J Biol Chem 1995;270:12953–6.

[25] Gerber P, Lubben G, Heusler S, et al. Effects of pioglitazone on metabolic control and blood pressure: a randomised study in patients with type 2 diabetes mellitus. Curr Med Res Opin 2003;19:532–9.

[26] van Wijk JP, de Koning EJ, Martens EP, et al. Thiazolidinediones and blood lipids in type 2 diabetes. Arterioscler Thromb Vasc Biol 2003;23:1744–9.

[27] Khan MA, St Peter JV, Xue JL. A prospective, randomized comparison of the metabolic effects of pioglitazone or rosiglitazone in patients with type 2 diabetes who were previously treated with troglitazone. Diabetes Care 2002;25:708–11.

[28] Li AC, Brown KK, Silvestre MJ, et al. Peroxisome proliferator-activated receptor gamma ligands inhibit development of atherosclerosis in LDL receptor-deficient mice. J Clin Invest 2000;106:523–31.

[29] Collins AR, Meehan WP, Kintscher U, et al. Troglitazone inhibits formation of early atherosclerotic lesions in diabetic and nondiabetic low density lipoprotein receptor-deficient mice. Arterioscler Thromb Vasc Biol 2001;21:365–71.

[30] Jiang C, Ting AT, Seed B. PPAR-gamma agonists inhibit production of monocyte inflammatory cytokines. Nature 1998;391:82–6.

[31] Pascual G, Fong AL, Ogawa S, et al. SUMOylation-dependent pathway mediates transrepression of inflammatory response genes by PPAR-gamma. Nature 2005;437: 759–63.

[32] Gearing KL, Gottlicher M, Teboul M, et al. Interaction of the peroxisome-proliferator-activated receptor and retinoid X receptor. Proc Natl Acad Sci USA 1993;90:1440–4.

[33] Tugwood JD, Issemann I, Anderson RG, et al. The mouse peroxisome proliferator activated receptor recognizes a response element in the 5′ flanking sequence of the rat acyl CoA oxidase gene. EMBO J 1992;11:433–9.

[34] Keller H, Dreyer C, Medin J, et al. Fatty acids and retinoids control lipid metabolism through activation of peroxisome proliferator-activated receptor-retinoid X receptor heterodimers. Proc Natl Acad Sci USA 1993;90:2160–4.

[35] Forman BM, Chen J, Evans RM. Hypolipidemic drugs, polyunsaturated fatty acids, and eicosanoids are ligands for peroxisome proliferator-activated receptors alpha and delta. Proc Natl Acad Sci USA 1997;94:4312–7.

[36] Krogsdam AM, Nielsen CA, Neve S, et al. Nuclear receptor corepressor-dependent repression of peroxisome-proliferator-activated receptor delta-mediated transactivation. Biochem J 2002;363:157–65.

[37] Li AC, Glass CK. PPAR- and LXR-dependent pathways controlling lipid metabolism and the development of atherosclerosis. J Lipid Res 2004;45:2161–73.

[38] Nolte RT, Wisely GB, Westin S, et al. Ligand binding and co-activator assembly of the peroxisome proliferator-activated receptor-gamma. Nature 1998;395:137–43.

[39] Ricote M, Li AC, Willson TM, et al. The peroxisome proliferator-activated receptor-gamma is a negative regulator of macrophage activation. Nature 1998;391:79–82.
[40] Ruan H, Lodish HF. Insulin resistance in adipose tissue: direct and indirect effects of tumor necrosis factor-alpha. Cytokine Growth Factor Rev 2003;14:447–55.
[41] Aizawa-Abe M, Ogawa Y, Masuzaki H, et al. Pathophysiological role of leptin in obesity-related hypertension. J Clin Invest 2000;105:1243–52.
[42] Yamauchi T, Kamon J, Ito Y, et al. Cloning of adiponectin receptors that mediate antidiabetic metabolic effects. Nature 2003;423:762–9.
[43] Yamauchi T, Kamon J, Waki H, et al. The fat-derived hormone adiponectin reverses insulin resistance associated with both lipoatrophy and obesity. Nat Med 2001;7:941–6.
[44] Yamauchi T, Kamon J, Minokoshi Y, et al. Adiponectin stimulates glucose utilization and fatty-acid oxidation by activating AMP-activated protein kinase. Nat Med 2002;8:1288–95.
[45] Chawla A, Schwarz EJ, Dimaculangan DD, et al. Peroxisome proliferator-activated receptor (PPAR) gamma: adipose-predominant expression and induction early in adipocyte differentiation. Endocrinology 1994;135:798–800.
[46] Tontonoz P, Hu E, Spiegelman BM. Regulation of adipocyte gene expression and differentiation by peroxisome proliferator activated receptor gamma. Curr Opin Genet Dev 1995;5:571–6.
[47] Tontonoz P, Hu E, Spiegelman BM. Stimulation of adipogenesis in fibroblasts by PPAR gamma 2, a lipid-activated transcription factor. Cell 1994;79:1147–56.
[48] Rosen ED, Sarraf P, Troy AE, et al. PPAR gamma is required for the differentiation of adipose tissue in vivo and in vitro. Mol Cell 1999;4:611–7.
[49] Kubota N, Terauchi Y, Miki H, et al. PPAR gamma mediates high-fat diet-induced adipocyte hypertrophy and insulin resistance. Mol Cell 1999;4:597–609.
[50] Zierath JR, Ryder JW, Doebber T, et al. Role of skeletal muscle in thiazolidinedione insulin sensitizer (PPARgamma agonist) action. Endocrinology 1998;139:5034–41.
[51] Kim SY, Kim HI, Park SK, et al. Liver glucokinase can be activated by peroxisome proliferator-activated receptor-gamma. Diabetes 2004;53(Suppl 1):S66–70.
[52] Chao L, Marcus-Samuels B, Mason MM, et al. Adipose tissue is required for the antidiabetic, but not for the hypolipidemic, effect of thiazolidinediones. J Clin Invest 2000;106:1221–8.
[53] Steppan CM, Bailey ST, Bhat S, et al. The hormone resistin links obesity to diabetes. Nature 2001;409:307–12.
[54] Marx N, Froehlich J, Siam L, et al. Antidiabetic PPAR gamma-activator rosiglitazone reduces MMP-9 serum levels in type 2 diabetic patients with coronary artery disease. Arterioscler Thromb Vasc Biol 2003;23:283–8.
[55] Maeda N, Takahashi M, Funahashi T, et al. PPARgamma ligands increase expression and plasma concentrations of adiponectin, an adipose-derived protein. Diabetes 2001;50:2094–9.
[56] Evans RM, Barish GD, Wang YX. PPARs and the complex journey to obesity. Nat Med 2004;10:355–61.
[57] Burant CF, Sreenan S, Hirano K, et al. Troglitazone action is independent of adipose tissue. J Clin Invest 1997;100:2900–8.
[58] Kim JK, Fillmore JJ, Gavrilova O, et al. Differential effects of rosiglitazone on skeletal muscle and liver insulin resistance in A-ZIP/F-1 fatless mice. Diabetes 2003;52:1311–8.
[59] Hevener AL, He W, Barak Y, et al. Muscle-specific Pparg deletion causes insulin resistance. Nat Med 2003;9:1491–7.
[60] Gavrilova O, Haluzik M, Matsusue K, et al. Liver peroxisome proliferator-activated receptor gamma contributes to hepatic steatosis, triglyceride clearance, and regulation of body fat mass. J Biol Chem 2003;278:34268–76.
[61] Norris AW, Chen L, Fisher SJ, et al. Muscle-specific PPARgamma-deficient mice develop increased adiposity and insulin resistance but respond to thiazolidinediones. J Clin Invest 2003;112:608–18.

[62] Marx N, Schonbeck U, Lazar MA, et al. Peroxisome proliferator-activated receptor gamma activators inhibit gene expression and migration in human vascular smooth muscle cells. Circ Res 1998;83:1097–103.

[63] Pasceri V, Wu HD, Willerson JT, et al. Modulation of vascular inflammation in vitro and in vivo by peroxisome proliferator-activated receptor-gamma activators. Circulation 2000; 101:235–8.

[64] Delerive P, Martin-Nizard F, Chinetti G, et al. Peroxisome proliferator-activated receptor activators inhibit thrombin-induced endothelin-1 production in human vascular endothelial cells by inhibiting the activator protein-1 signaling pathway. Circ Res 1999;85:394–402.

[65] Marx N, Mach F, Sauty A, et al. Peroxisome proliferator-activated receptor-gamma activators inhibit IFN-gamma-induced expression of the T cell-active CXC chemokines IP-10, Mig, and I-TAC in human endothelial cells. J Immunol 2000;164:6503–8.

[66] Oyama Y, Akuzawa N, Nagai R, et al. PPARgamma ligand inhibits osteopontin gene expression through interference with binding of nuclear factors to A/T-rich sequence in THP-1 cells. Circ Res 2002;90:348–55.

[67] Takata Y, Kitami Y, Yang ZH, et al. Vascular inflammation is negatively autoregulated by interaction between CCAAT/enhancer-binding protein-delta and peroxisome proliferator-activated receptor-gamma. Circ Res 2002;91:427–33.

[68] Ruan H, Pownall HJ, Lodish HF. Troglitazone antagonizes tumor necrosis factor-alpha-induced reprogramming of adipocyte gene expression by inhibiting the transcriptional regulatory functions of NF-kappaB. J Biol Chem 2003;278:28181–92.

[69] Su CG, Wen X, Bailey ST, et al. A novel therapy for colitis utilizing PPAR-gamma ligands to inhibit the epithelial inflammatory response. J Clin Invest 1999;104:383–9.

[70] Chawla A, Barak Y, Nagy L, et al. PPAR-gamma dependent and independent effects on macrophage-gene expression in lipid metabolism and inflammation. Nat Med 2001;7: 48–52.

[71] Claudel T, Leibowitz MD, Fievet C, et al. Reduction of atherosclerosis in apolipoprotein E knockout mice by activation of the retinoid X receptor. Proc Natl Acad Sci USA 2001;98: 2610–5.

[72] Chen Z, Ishibashi S, Perrey S, et al. Troglitazone inhibits atherosclerosis in apolipoprotein E-knockout mice: pleiotropic effects on CD36 expression and HDL. Arterioscler Thromb Vasc Biol 2001;21:372–7.

[73] Kintscher U, Lyon CJ, LawAngiotensin RE II. PPAR-gamma and atherosclerosis. Front Biosci 2004;9:359–69.

[74] Goetze S, Xi XP, Kawano H, et al. PPAR gamma-ligands inhibit migration mediated by multiple chemoattractants in vascular smooth muscle cells. J Cardiovasc Pharmacol 1999;33:798–806.

[75] Wakino S, Kintscher U, Kim S, et al. Peroxisome proliferator-activated receptor gamma ligands inhibit retinoblastoma phosphorylation and G1 → S transition in vascular smooth muscle cells. J Biol Chem 2000;275:22435–41.

[76] Kintscher U, Goetze S, Wakino S, et al. Peroxisome proliferator-activated receptor and retinoid X receptor ligands inhibit monocyte chemotactic protein-1-directed migration of monocytes. Eur J Pharmacol 2000;401:259–70.

[77] Takeda K, Ichiki T, Tokunou T, et al. Peroxisome proliferator-activated receptor gamma activators downregulate angiotensin II type 1 receptor in vascular smooth muscle cells. Circulation 2000;102:1834–9.

[78] Goetze S, Xi XP, Graf K, et al. Troglitazone inhibits angiotensin II-induced extracellular signal-regulated kinase 1/2 nuclear translocation and activation in vascular smooth muscle cells. FEBS Lett 1999;452:277–82.

[79] Tontonoz P, Nagy L, Alvarez JG, et al. PPARgamma promotes monocyte/macrophage differentiation and uptake of oxidized LDL. Cell 1998;93:241–52.

[80] Nagy L, Tontonoz P, Alvarez JG, et al. Oxidized LDL regulates macrophage gene expression through ligand activation of PPARgamma. Cell 1998;93:229–40.

[81] Chawla A, Boisvert WA, Lee CH, et al. PPAR gamma-LXR-ABCA1 pathway in macrophages is involved in cholesterol efflux and atherogenesis. Mol Cell 2001;7:161–71.

[82] Li AC, Binder CJ, Gutierrez A, et al. Differential inhibition of macrophage foam-cell formation and atherosclerosis in mice by PPARalpha, beta/delta, and gamma. J Clin Invest 2004;114:1564–76.

[83] Wang N, Lan D, Chen W, et al. ATP-binding cassette transporters G1 and G4 mediate cellular cholesterol efflux to high-density lipoproteins. Proc Natl Acad Sci USA 2004; 101:9774–9.

[84] Dormandy JA, Charbonnel B, Eckland DJ, et al. Secondary prevention of macrovascular events in patients with type 2 diabetes in the PROactive Study (PROspective pioglitAzone Clinical Trial In macroVascular Events): a randomised controlled trial. Lancet 2005;366: 1279–89.

[85] Minamikawa J, Tanaka S, Yamauchi M, et al. Potent inhibitory effect of troglitazone on carotid arterial wall thickness in type 2 diabetes. J Clin Endocrinol Metab 1998;83: 1818–20.

[86] Koshiyama H, Shimono D, Kuwamura N, et al. Rapid communication: inhibitory effect of pioglitazone on carotid arterial wall thickness in type 2 diabetes. J Clin Endocrinol Metab 2001;86:3452–6.

[87] Quinones MJ, Hernandez-Pampaloni M, Schelbert H, et al. Coronary vasomotor abnormalities in insulin-resistant individuals. Ann Intern Med 2004;140:700–8.

[88] Haffner SM, Greenberg AS, Weston WM, et al. Effect of rosiglitazone treatment on nontraditional markers of cardiovascular disease in patients with type 2 diabetes mellitus. Circulation 2002;106:679–84.

[89] Satoh N, Ogawa Y, Usui T, et al. Antiatherogenic effect of pioglitazone in type 2 diabetic patients irrespective of the responsiveness to its antidiabetic effect. Diabetes Care 2003;26: 2493–9.

[90] Kruszynska YT, Yu JG, Olefsky JM, et al. Effects of troglitazone on blood concentrations of plasminogen activator inhibitor 1 in patients with type 2 diabetes and in lean and obese normal subjects. Diabetes 2000;49:633–9.

[91] Raskin P, Rappaport EB, Cole ST, et al. Rosiglitazone short-term monotherapy lowers fasting and post-prandial glucose in patients with type II diabetes. Diabetologia 2000;43: 278–84.

[92] Festa A, D'Agostino R Jr, Mykkanen L, et al. Relative contribution of insulin and its precursors to fibrinogen and PAI-1 in a large population with different states of glucose tolerance. The Insulin Resistance Atherosclerosis Study (IRAS). Arterioscler Thromb Vasc Biol 1999;19:562–8.

[93] Thogersen AM, Jansson JH, Boman K, et al. High plasminogen activator inhibitor and tissue plasminogen activator levels in plasma precede a first acute myocardial infarction in both men and women: evidence for the fibrinolytic system as an independent primary risk factor. Circulation 1998;98:2241–7.

[94] Schwartz SM, Liaw L. Growth control and morphogenesis in the development and pathology of arteries. J Cardiovasc Pharmacol 1993;21(Suppl 1):S31–49.

[95] Dzau VJ, Braun-Dullaeus RC, Sedding DG. Vascular proliferation and atherosclerosis: new perspectives and therapeutic strategies. Nat Med 2002;8:1249–56.

[96] The BARI Investigators. Seven-year outcome in the Bypass Angioplasty Revascularization Investigation (BARI) by treatment and diabetic status. J Am Coll Cardiol 2000;35:1122–9.

[97] Harbour JW, Dean DC. Rb function in cell-cycle regulation and apoptosis. Nat Cell Biol 2000;2:E65–7.

[98] Weinberg RA. E2F and cell proliferation: a world turned upside down. Cell 1996;85:457–9.

[99] Goetze S, Kintscher U, Kim S, et al. Peroxisome proliferator-activated receptor-gamma ligands inhibit nuclear but not cytosolic extracellular signal-regulated kinase/mitogen-activated protein kinase-regulated steps in vascular smooth muscle cell migration. J Cardiovasc Pharmacol 2001;38:909–21.

[100] Desouza CV, Murthy SN, Diez J, et al. Differential effects of peroxisome proliferator acti- vator receptor-alpha and gamma ligands on intimal hyperplasia after balloon catheter- induced vascular injury in Zucker rats. J Cardiovasc Pharmacol Ther 2003;8:297–305.

[101] Yoshimoto T, Naruse M, Shizume H, et al. Vasculo-protective effects of insulin sensitizing agent pioglitazone in neointimal thickening and hypertensive vascular hypertrophy. Ath- erosclerosis 1999;145:333–40.

[102] Takagi T, Yamamuro A, Tamita K, et al. Pioglitazone reduces neointimal tissue prolifer- ation after coronary stent implantation in patients with type 2 diabetes mellitus: an intra- vascular ultrasound scanning study. Am Heart J 2003;146:E5.

[103] Choi D, Kim SK, Choi SH, et al. Preventative effects of rosiglitazone on restenosis after coronary stent implantation in patients with type 2 diabetes. Diabetes Care 2004;27: 2654–60.

[104] American Heart Association. . Heart and Stroke facts: 2002 statistical supplement. Dallas (TX): American Heart Association; 2002.

[105] Mudaliar S, Chang AR, Henry RR. Thiazolidinediones, peripheral edema, and type 2 di- abetes: incidence, pathophysiology, and clinical implications. Endocr Pract 2003;9:406–16.

[106] Avandia prescribing information. Research Triangle Park (NC): GlaxoSmithKline; 2003.

[107] Actos prescribing information. Lincolnshire (IL): Takeda Pharmaceuticals America, Inc; 2003.

[108] Nesto RW, Bell D, Bonow RO, et al. Thiazolidinedione use, fluid retention, and congestive heart failure: a consensus statement from the American Heart Association and American Diabetes Association. October 7, 2003. Circulation 2003;108:2941–8.

[109] Lefebvre AM, Chen I, Desreumaux P, et al. Activation of the peroxisome proliferator- activated receptor gamma promotes the development of colon tumors in C57BL/6J- APCMin/ + mice. Nat Med 1998;4:1053–7.

[110] Sarraf P, Mueller E, Jones D, et al. Differentiation and reversal of malignant changes in colon cancer through PPARgamma. Nat Med 1998;4:1046–52.

ELSEVIER
SAUNDERS

Endocrinol Metab Clin N Am
35 (2006) 575–599

ENDOCRINOLOGY
AND METABOLISM
CLINICS
OF NORTH AMERICA

Diabetic Cardiomyopathy

Gregg C. Fonarow, MD[a],*, Preethi Srikanthan, MD[b]

[a]*Ahmanson–UCLA Cardiomyopathy Center, UCLA Division of Cardiology,
David Geffen School of Medicine at UCLA, 10833 Leconte Avenue,
Room BH407, Los Angeles, CA 90095, USA*
[b]*Division of Epidemiology and Preventative Medicine,
David Geffen School of Medicine at UCLA, Box 957065, 330 South Garfield Avenue,
Suite 308, Los Angeles, CA 90095, USA*

Cardiomyopathy is defined as disease of the myocardium associated with cardiac dysfunction. The World Health Organization guidelines on the definition and classification of cardiomyopathy were revised in 1996 to reflect the insight gained into the pathogenesis of heart muscle disorders [1]. Cardiomyopathies are divided into those that are intrinsic or specific to the myocardium: *Intrinsic* cardiomyopathies are based on the predominant pathophysiologic characteristics that are manifest, and *specific* cardiomyopathies are associated with distinct systemic or cardiac diseases (ischemic, valvular, hypertensive, and diabetic cardiomyopathy).

Diabetes, which has steadily increased in prevalence (from 4% of the population in 1995 to an estimated 5.4% in 2025) [2], is strongly associated with cardiovascular disease. The 7-year incidence of myocardial infarction in diabetics (with no previous myocardial infarction) is 20.2% compared with only 3.5% in a similar population of nondiabetics [3]. Two thirds of the 16 million diabetic patients in the United States are expected to die of some form of heart or blood vessel disease, of which coronary artery disease is the most common cardiac manifestation. Heart failure not of ischemic origin is also a significant source of morbidity and mortality. The Framingham Heart Study determined that the relative risk of congestive heart failure is approximately two times as high for men with diabetes and five times as high for women with diabetes compared with the general population [4].

Diabetic cardiomyopathy (DCM) may be characterized functionally by ventricular dilation, myocyte hypertrophy, prominent interstitial fibrosis, and decreased or preserved systolic function. Postulated etiologies include

---

* Corresponding author.
E-mail address: gfonarow@mednet.uca.edu (G.C. Fonarow).

0889-8529/06/$ - see front matter © 2006 Elsevier Inc. All rights reserved.
doi:10.1016/j.ecl.2006.05.003   *endo.theclinics.com*

(1) *microangiopathy,* related to endothelial dysfunction; (2) *autonomic neuropathy,* as a complication of diabetes; and (3) *metabolic factors,* such as abnormal myocardial use of glucose predisposing to inappropriate response to ischemia and other cardiac stress. Heart failure can result in the presence of preserved systolic function secondary to impaired ventricular relaxation and filling or a fibrotic process involving myocytes and the cardiac interstitium (diastolic dysfunction) or both. Increased diastolic myocardial stiffness in the presence of normal left ventricular systolic function and mass is the earliest discernible evidence of DCM. Even quite early in the course of the metabolic derangements of diabetes, 50% to 60% of diabetic patients have been reported to show some degree of diastolic abnormality in community studies and clinical trials [5–8]. Heart failure also may result from systolic dysfunction owing to reduced cardiac output, increased atrioventricular valvular regurgitation, and the resulting peripheral responses. Studies have observed significantly reduced left ventricular systolic function in diabetic compared with nondiabetic individuals [9] and a correlation between systolic function and glycemic control [10,11].

Several distinct pathologic processes may initiate myocyte injury, ventricular dilation, and myocardial dysfunction in patients with diabetes. Common pathophysiologic pathways are activated when a certain level of injury and myocardial dysfunction has occurred, regardless of the initial myocardial insult or process that initiated the cardiomyopathy. These common pathways involve neurohumoral and other growth factors, cytokines, immune factors, and oxidative stress. These pathways contribute to progressive myocyte dysfunction, cell loss, and ventricular dilation that result in further disease progression. As the disease progresses, cardiac function deteriorates so that patients exhibit characteristic symptoms of heart failure. Patients manifest cardiac and extracardiac signs and symptoms that are not specific to the underlying etiology of the cardiomyopathy. Severe heart failure or sudden cardiac death results if the pathophysiologic processes set in motion are not interrupted. This article focuses on more recent advances in the understanding of the pathogenesis and treatment of DCM.

Diabetes and the risk of heart failure

Pathophysiology of diabetic cardiomyopathy: metabolic derangements

In the 1950s, Ungar and coworkers [12] recognized that cardiac myocytes from a patient with diabetes have abnormal, energy-inefficient metabolic function. In an assessment of coronary sinus blood samples from diabetic patients, there was a significant decline in myocardial glucose, pyruvate, and lactate consumption, whereas there was an increase in fatty acid extraction and storage. The changes in metabolism resemble the changes in ischemia, where there is (1) decreased myocardial glucose uptake and glucose oxidation and (2) increased fatty oxidation with subsequent inhibition of pyruvate dehydrogenase activity. Ungar and coworkers [12] surmised that the chief abnormality in myocytes from diabetics related to the inability of the myocardium to metabolize pyruvate, and in the presence of an energy deficit (as in ischemia), the myocyte sustained reperfusion injuries. Pyruvate is a product of glycolysis, and with its accumulation, glycolytic flux is inhibited, and a greater fraction of the glucose uptake and glucose-6-phosphate is directed toward glycogen synthesis. Glycolytically derived ATP is preferentially used for Ca^{2+} reuptake into the sarcoplasmic reticulum, which is why it is essential for optimal diastolic function. Evidence for this concept comes from studies in isolated tissues showing that inhibition of glycolysis resulted in impaired relaxation, especially in ischemic or reperfused myocardiums, and may result in cardiac hypertrophy.

Additionally, diabetes is associated with hyperglycemia, insulin resistance, and increased free fatty acid. These metabolic changes result in biochemical events that produce cardiomyopathy (Figs. 1 and 2) [13,14]. The core defect in type 2 diabetes is insulin resistance leading to compensatory hyperinsulinemia and eventually hyperglycemia [15]. Festa and colleagues [16] found that fasting insulin, intact proinsulin, split proinsulin, insulin sensitivity, and insulin secretion are significantly associated with heart rate, supporting the link between heart rate, hyperinsulinemia, and sympathetic nervous system activation. Elevated resting heart rate has been shown to be a risk factor for death from coronary heart disease [17,18]. Hyperinsulinemia is associated with increased free fatty acid levels in diabetic patients, and activation of the sympathetic nervous system in diabetic patients results in increased myocardial use of free fatty acids. The myocardial response to the diabetic environment consists of cardiac myocyte hypertrophy, myocardial ischemia, reduced cardiac function, cardiac arrhythmias, interstitial fibrosis, and intracellular triglyceride accumulation secondary to increased

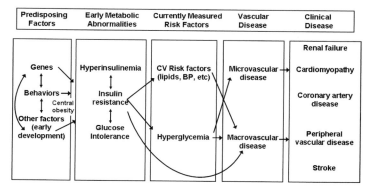

Fig. 1. Pathophysiologic model of development of diabetes and vascular/cardiovascular (CV) disease. BP, blood pressure. (*Adapted from* Howard BV, Rodriguez BL, Bennett PH, et al. Prevention Conference VI: diabetes and cardiovascular disease. Writing Group I: epidemiology. Circulation 2002;105:e132–7; with permission.)

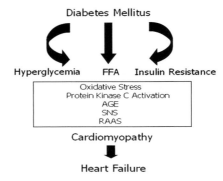

Fig. 2. Diabetes leading to cardiomyopathy and heart failure. This figure shows the contribution of diabetes/insulin resistance to heart injury and activation of the renin-angiotensin-aldosterone system (RAAS) and sympathetic nervous system (SNS). AGE, advanced glycosylation end product; FFA, free fatty acid. (*Adapted from* Giles TD, Sander GE. Diabetes mellitus and heart failure: basic mechanisms, clinical features, and therapeutic considerations. Cardiol Clin 2004;22:553–68; with permission.)

fatty acid uptake [19,20]. Increased levels of insulin have been thought to promote cellular hypertrophy by binding to the insulin-like growth factor-1 receptor owing to the similarities in its extracellular domain with the insulin receptor, although binding occurs with a 100-fold lower affinity [21]. In humans, insulin has been shown to reduce protein degradation in the heart without affecting net protein synthesis, also potentially contributing to myocardial hypertrophy [22]. In addition, chronic hyperinsulinemia may promote afterload-stimulated left ventricular hypertrophy by increasing sympathetic nervous system activity; in contrast to hepatic, skeletal muscle, cardiac, and adipose tissue, the sympathetic nervous system remains insulin-sensitive in the presence of diabetes [23]. Heart failure itself can intensify insulin resistance via enhanced neurohumoral activation that accompanies cardiac decompensation [24].

Changes of diabetic cardiomyopathy have been noted in type 1 and type 2 diabetes, as illustrated by parallel changes in animal models, OVE26 and db/db mice [25]. Both diabetic models show significant impairment in cardiac contractility. There is a difference in myocyte calcium reuptake rate, however, which is likely to be related to differences in sarcoplasmic reticulum calcium-ATPase (SERCA2) concentration, which are due to differences in the expression of the antioxidant protein metallothionein and related oxidative stress.

Diastolic dysfunction associated with DCM is primarily due to quantitative and qualitative changes in interstitial collagen [26]. In experimental models of early diabetes and impaired fasting glucose, hyperglycemia is associated with increased myocardial stiffness as a result of the accumulation of advanced glycosylation end products (AGEs) bound onto collagen, even before the increase in intracellular matrix protein [27,28]. In older animals, these changes also are accompanied by an increase in collagen I and III protein content [29]. In the presence of chronic hyperglycemia, collagen becomes irreversibly associated through nonenzymatic glycosylation with AGEs, which form covalent crosslinks throughout the collagen molecule, serving as the major source of increased myocardial stiffness [30]. Strong evidence for the role of crosslinked collagen AGEs in DCM is provided by studies showing that treating animal models of diabetes or impaired fasting glucose with agents that block (aminoguanidine) or break (phenyl-4, 5-dimethylthazolium chloride [ALT-711]) AGE crosslinkages prevented or reversed myocardial stiffness [27,28].

AGEs also may promote fibrosis through specific AGE cell surface receptors that increase expression of prosclerotic cytokines. Diabetic mice show increased protein expression of connective tissue growth factor in left ventricular tissue [31]. Animal models of early diabetic heart disease have exhibited coronary arteriolar perivascular fibrosis and increased wall-to-lumen ratio, which may contribute an ischemic component to the myocardial abnormalities of DCM [32].

Hyperglycemia induces the production of reactive nitrogen and oxygen species, leading to oxidative myocardial injury. The heart is a susceptible target because it contains low levels of free radical scavengers. The reactive nitrogen and oxygen species cause an increase in mitochondrial superoxide anion production, glucose auto-oxidation, and cardiac lipid peroxidation on exposure to an oxidative stress. Oxidative stress results in abnormal gene expression, altered signal transduction, and activation of pathways leading to programmed myocardial cell death [33]. A transgenic mouse model with overexpression of an antioxidant protein (metallothionein) specifically in the heart has been produced [34]. When this mouse was crossed with a model of type 1 diabetes (OVE26), the resultant mouse had significant improvement in the myocardial morphologic changes compared with that seen in OVE26 myocardium, which had collections of mitochondria that were interspersed randomly between disrupted myofibrils in an edematous sarcoplasm, and with numerous myelin figures suggesting membrane disruption and cellular damage. There also was altered mRNA expression and increased oxidized glutathione indicating oxidative stress, whereas the myocytes had reduced contractility under ischemic conditions. These changes were reversed in the OVE26/metallothionein mouse.

In diabetic cardiomyopathy, there is an alteration in contractile proteins and the electromechanical milieu as a result of changes in calcium transport in the sarcoplasmic reticulum, all of which result in altered cardiac contractility. Changes in protein kinase C can cause changes in myocardial contractility. Protein kinase C has been shown to inhibit myofibrillar ATPase by phosphorylation of troponin T and I, and it phosphorylates phospholamban, inhibiting calcium uptake. Liu and coworkers [35] showed changes in protein kinase C isoenzymes in cardiac homogenate from rats, followed over 8 weeks after induction of diabetes by streptozocin. The activity of protein kinase C was increased at 4 weeks (70%) and at 8 weeks (89%). This increase was partially reversible on treatment of the diabetic rats with insulin. This change in calcium metabolism in diabetes has been shown to alter cardiac metabolism. During diastole, myocardial oxygen consumption per beat is principally used for calcium handling during the excitation-contraction coupling, especially the activity of SERCA2 [36]. In Otsuka Long-Evans Tokushima Fatty (OLETF) mouse model of type 2 diabetes, diastolic dysfunction manifested itself with a depressed SERCA2 protein and a decrease in myocardial oxygen consumption per beat during diastole (presumably owing to lack of SERCA2 activity [36]). AGEs, acting through their receptors, trigger intracellular signals involving mitogen-activated protein kinase and $P21^{ras}$, which cause impaired calcium homeostasis secondary to a decline in SERCA2, phospholambin, and the Na^+-Ca^{2+} exchanger quantity [37]. In the myocardium of rats with alloxan-induced diabetes, there was a depression in the Na^+-Ca^{2+} exchange and ATP-dependent Ca^{2+} uptake within 2 weeks after diabetes induction. This change correlated with a decline in the Na^+-K^+ ATPase α_1-subunit mRNA content in these myocardiums [37]. Na^+-Ca^{2+} activity decline leads to intracellular calcium overload, which results in contractile failure, and eventually development of DCM. The Na^+-Ca^{2+} activities were normalized on treatment of diabetic animals with insulin. Voltage clamps on guinea pig atrial myocytes showed that troglitazone-inhibited calcium L-type and T-type voltage-dependent channels, playing a role in prevention of diabetes-induced intracellular calcium overload and subsequent development of DCM [38].

There is frequently a prolonged action potential duration in myocytes from diabetics, which is likely to be important in the development of diastolic dysfunction because it results in delayed repolarization. Delayed repolarization also is the result of decreased outward potassium currents, and a variety of potassium currents have been noted to have such modulatory effects. The repolarization of the myocardium after an action potential is governed by the activity of potassium channels through potassium currents (I_{Ks}, I_{Kr}, I_{K1}), each differing in voltage at activation and duration of activation properties [39]. The calcium-independent transient outward current I_{to} is consistently decreased in cardiac disorders, such as DCM, in which there is electrical remodeling. DCM causes alterations in transcription and surface expression of potassium channel proteins, which are theorized to be under the control of the insulin-signaling cascade. Pyruvate dehydrogenase is a multienzyme complex on the inner mitochondrial membrane that converts pyruvate into acetyl coenzyme A. Its activation (by insulin) upregulates I_{to} channels, and they are generally downregulated in diabetes. Similar potassium channel remodeling in the myocardium also occurs after oxidative stress [39]. Such electrical remodeling is hypothesized to favor the genesis of lethal arrhythmias in the diabetic myocardium; it also exacerbates the progression to contractile failure secondary to delayed repolarization and prolongation of the intracellular calcium concentration and the action potential.

A metabolic hypothesis has been proposed to explain the progression of DCM from early diastolic abnormalities to contractile dysfunction [40]. In the early insulin-resistant state, intracellular fatty acids are increased, whereas glucose is regulated by compensatory hyperglycemia. The cardiac myocyte responds to increased fatty acid levels by upregulating the expression of the enzymes necessary for their disposal through mitochondrial β-oxidation. These enzymes are under the transcriptional control of the nuclear transcription factor peroxisome proliferator-activated receptor-α (PPARα). PPARα downregulation seems to be important in insulin-resistant states and in type 2 diabetes per se. PPARα null mice, subjected to long-term high-fat feeding, developed a twofold rise in blood lipids, yet remained normoglycemic and normoinsulinemic—showing that the absence of PPARα influences insulin resistance, despite its effect on blood lipids [41]. In states of chronic hyperglycemia, glucose downregulates PPARα, resulting in promotion of lipid esterification and triglyceride cellular deposition [42]. Cardiac myocytes consequently are unable to metabolize their increased fatty acid load, which leads to accumulated intracellular lipids. This accumulation can result in increased nonoxidative production of ceramide, a toxic lipid product. Increased ceramide levels in the cardiac myocyte are associated with increased oxidative stress, apoptosis, and decreased contractile function [40]. In mice with cardiac restricted overexpression of PPARα, glucose uptake and use in the heart were decreased, whereas myocardial fatty acid oxidation increased and features of diabetic cardiomyopathy, such as ventricular hypertrophy, were noted [43]. Another transgenic animal producing myocardial changes of diabetic cardiomyopathy was that produced by Yagyu and colleagues [44], in which an α-myosin heavy-chain promoter was placed upstream of a human lipoprotein lipase minigene construct, with the resulting transgenic mice expressing the altered lipoprotein lipase on the surface of cardiomyocytes. Hearts of the transgenic mice had greater lipid accumulation, were dilated, and had impaired left ventricular systolic function. In an experimental animal model of diabetes marked by intracellular triglyceride accumulation, high ceramide levels, and apoptosis, the PPARγ agonist troglitazone (which at high concentrations is an agonist of PPARα) reduced myocardial triglycerides, ceramide, and evidence of apoptosis, while preserving normal contractile function [45].

Other mechanisms for development of myocardial dysfunction in type 2 diabetes

Microangiopathy
The pathologic evidence that first described the phenomenon of microangiopathy included subendothelial and endothelial fibrosis and endothelial proliferation with periodic acid–Schiff–positive material in 50% of patients with diabetes compared with 21% of nondiabetics [46]. More recent studies

have linked the hyperglycemic milieu and AGE proteins in the extracellular matrix of microvasculature in an animal model [47]. The functional significance of such lesions as a primary pathology has been questioned, however, after studies by Regan and coworkers [48] in which patients with diabetes who underwent angiograms had no epicardial disease and no evidence of lactate production on coronary venous sinus sampling, suggesting no evidence of functionally significant microvasculature disease. Similarly, Moir and associates [49] noted in a study of type 2 diabetics that quantitative myocardial contrast echocardiogram showed impaired myocardial blood flow reserve; however, this did not correlate with subclinical longitudinal myocardial dysfunction.

Autonomic neuropathy

Catecholamines modulate the contractility of cardiac myocytes through facilitation of sarcoplasmic reticulum calcium uptake. Dysregulation of autonomic innervation of the myocardium has been noted to contribute to myocardial dysfunction and potentially increased cardiac mortality in diabetes. The mechanism by which changes in myocardial autonomic innervation results in myocardial dysfunction involves alteration in diurnal variation in blood pressure. The normal 24-hour variation in blood pressure and echocardiographic function in 19 patients with type 1 diabetes (8 with autonomic neuropathy) was less pronounced in the patients with autonomic neuropathy, resulting in a higher ambient blood pressure for longer periods during the day, predisposing to hypertension-induced left ventricular changes [5]. It has been noted that the mean serum catecholamine concentration in patients with long-standing diabetes is 6% to 20% of population control values. Correspondingly, I^{125}MIBG (an analogue of norepinephrine) scanning has shown denervation in the hearts of diabetic patients with autonomic neuropathy, which corresponds to the echocardiographic and radionuclide ventriculograms, as evidence of diastolic dysfunction [5,50]. Such an association between diastolic dysfunction and autonomic neuropathy has been noted by several groups, with 59% of patients with diabetes who had autonomic dysfunction having abnormal diastolic function compared with 8% of patients with diabetes but without autonomic neuropathy [51]. Most importantly, the development of autonomic neuropathy results in a decline in survival in patients with diabetes, from 85% to 44% [52].

Other mechanisms have been postulated for the deterioration of systolic function in DCM, including ischemia from microvascular disease or dysregulation, altered myocardial energy metabolism, activation of protein kinase $C–\beta_2$ activity by hyperglycemia with subsequent myocardial necrosis and fibrosis, and hyperglycemia-induced increases in oxidative stress. This leads to a wide variety of potentially harmful responses, including myocardial inflammation, defective calcium transport, mitochondrial dysfunction, and apoptosis [26,40,53].

Final common pathway of neurohumoral activation

Neurohumoral and other growth factors, cytokines, immune factors, and oxidative stress contribute to progressive myocyte dysfunction, cell loss, and ventricular dilation that result in further disease progression. Activation of the sympathetic nervous system and the renin-angiotensin-aldosterone system is a fundamental pathophysiologic abnormality in patients with chronic heart failure [24]. Activation of the sympathetic nervous system is defined mainly by increased plasma levels of catecholamines (eg, norepinephrine), and higher levels indicate a worse prognosis. The deleterious effects of norepinephrine on the heart and circulation include cardiac myocyte death and dysfunction, increased ventricular size and pressures, proarrhythmic effects, and increased heart rate [24]. Myocardial injury also activates the renin-angiotensin-aldosterone system. This results in prolonged expression of angiotensin II, which increases blood pressure by increasing total peripheral resistance and inhibiting sodium excretion. Long-term effects of angiotensin II include vascular and cardiac hypertrophy and remodeling, which are primary factors in the progression of heart failure and mortality [54].

Diabetes and the mechanics of heart failure

Heart failure affects nearly 5 million Americans, and related deaths total 300,000 each year; related deaths and hospitalizations have increased steadily over the past several years despite advances in treatment [55]. As noted, since the time of the Framingham Heart Study 2 decades ago, it has been known that patients with diabetes have a particularly increased risk of heart failure [4]. More recent data from the Acute Decompensated Heart Failure National Registry (ADHERE) show that approximately 44% of patients hospitalized with acutely decompensated heart failure have diabetes mellitus [56]. Community and retrospective studies and clinical trials have confirmed that patients with diabetes have a higher prevalence and risk for congestive heart failure than their nondiabetic counterparts [57]. In addition, studies have established that each 1% increase in hemoglobin A_{1c} levels is significantly and linearly associated with an increasing risk of developing heart failure in all patients, with a 15% increase in the incidence of heart failure for every 1% increase in hemoglobin A_{1c} ($P = .009$) [58]. A report on more than 48,000 patients with diabetes from the Kaiser Permanente Medical Care Program found that every 1% increase in hemoglobin A_{1c} was associated with a 12% increase in the risk of new-onset heart failure over a 2.2-year follow-up period [59]. A review of nationwide hospital discharge data reported that diabetic patients had a ninefold higher discharge diagnosis of idiopathic cardiomyopathy [60]. Similarly, the United Kingdom Prospective Diabetes Study (UKPDS) reported that the incidence of heart failure increased from 2.3 to 11.9 cases per 1000 person-years for hemoglobin A_{1c} levels less than 6% compared with levels 10% or greater [61].

The American College of Cardiology/American Heart Association (ACC/AHA) classifies DCM as stage A heart failure owing to the role that it plays in the development and progression of the disease (Table 1) [55]. Stage A patients have a structurally normal heart and no heart failure symptoms, but are at high risk of developing heart failure as a result of diabetes, hypertension, coronary artery disease, or a family history of cardiomyopathy [8,62]. The earliest discernible evidence of DCM is an increase in diastolic myocardial stiffness detected clinically by Doppler echocardiography in the presence of normal left ventricular systolic function and mass. Left ventricular diastolic dysfunction (LVDD) is indicated by a decreased rate of early diastolic filling, a compensatory increase in atrial filling velocity (decreased early-to-late ratio), and a prolongation of isovolumetric relaxation [5]. In a study of asymptomatic, normotensive, well-controlled type 2 diabetic patients, the average early-to-late peak flow ratio was 22% lower, early peak filling rate was 24% lower, and early acceleration peak was 23% lower than in matched control subjects [53]. Studies have found significant increases in left ventricular wall thickness and left ventricular mass in patients with diabetes compared with nondiabetic individuals [9], and the incidence of LVDD in patient populations with well-controlled type 2 diabetes without hypertension, structural heart disease, or congestive heart failure has been reported to be 50% to 60% [6,7].

Table 1
Approach to the classification of heart failure: American College of Cardiology/American Heart Association heart failure guidelines

Stage	Patient description
A: High risk for developing heart failure	Hypertension Coronary artery disease Diabetes mellitus Family history of cardiomyopathy
B: Asymptomatic left ventricular dysfunction	Previous myocardial infarction Left ventricular systolic dysfunction Asymptomatic valvular disease
C: Symptomatic left ventricular dysfunction	Known structural heart disease Shortness of breath and fatigue Reduced exercise tolerance
D: Refractory end-stage heart failure	Marked symptoms at rest despite maximal medical therapy (eg, Patients who are recurrently hospitalized or cannot be safely discharged from the hospital without specialized interventions)

From Hunt SA, Baker DW, Chin MH, et al. ACC/AHA guidelines for the evaluation and management of chronic heart failure in the adult: executive summary. A report of the American College of Cardiology/American Heart Association Task Force on Practice Guidelines (Committee to revise the 1995 Guidelines for the Evaluation and Management of Heart Failure). J Am Coll Cardiol 2001;38:2101–13; with permission.

Left ventricular systolic dysfunction (LVSD) also may be encountered frequently in the diabetic population, although it generally occurs later in the natural history of diabetes (Fig. 3) [62,63]. Large studies have observed significantly reduced echocardiographic parameters of left ventricular systolic function in patients with diabetes compared with matched nondiabetic individuals [9]. Factors associated with insulin resistance, such as proinsulin levels, in individuals with no heart disease predicts LVSD (ejection fraction <40%) years later [64]. Evidence of subtle systolic dysfunction also has been reported as an early manifestation of DCM in diabetic patients with no overt cardiac disease in whom the left ventricular ejection fraction was still greater than 50% and was inversely related to the degree of glycemic control [65].

Clinical presentation of diabetic cardiomyopathy

DCM may have a long asymptomatic period, especially in patients with type 2 diabetes, and its earliest presentation often may be due to concomitant hypertension or coronary heart disease. The LVDD of early DCM is associated with only mild effects on ventricular filling as shown by Doppler echocardiography in most cases (80%), whereas physiologic restriction is an uncommon finding (3%) [66]. The subsequent presentation of systolic dysfunction is indistinguishable from other dilated cardiomyopathies with variable symptoms of congestive heart failure, including exertional dyspnea, orthopnea, effort intolerance, early fatigability, and peripheral edema. Patients with diabetes who have clinical heart failure and patients with asymptomatic LVSD have been found to have significantly worse outcomes, however, including myocardial infarction, angina, pulmonary edema,

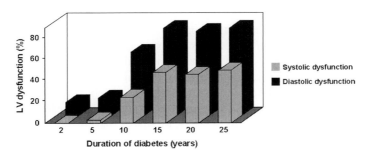

Fig. 3. Frequency distribution of left ventricular (LV) dysfunction in diabetics depending on the duration of diabetes. LV dysfunction is significantly more frequent with longer duration of diabetes ($P < .001$), and diastolic dysfunction is more frequent than systolic. The presence of systolic dysfunction is not apparent until 10 years after diagnosis of diabetes. (*Adapted from* Raev DC. Which left ventricular function is impaired earlier in the evolution of diabetic cardiomyopathy? An echocardiographic study of young type I diabetic patients. Diabetes Care 1994;17:633–9; with permission.)

hospitalization for heart failure, and death, than control-matched nondiabetics [67].

An asymptomatic diabetic patient may show subtle signs of DCM related to decreased left ventricular compliance or left ventricular hypertrophy or both. Physical examination may show prominence of an "a" wave in the jugular venous pulse, and the cardiac apical impulse may be overactive or sustained throughout systole, rather than tapping normally. Auscultation may reveal a fourth heart sound. After the development of systolic dysfunction, left ventricular dilation, and symptomatic heart failure, the jugular venous pressure may become elevated, the apical impulse would be displaced downward and to the left, and a third heart sound and a systolic mitral valve murmur may be heard. Several studies have documented a variety of electrocardiographic changes that may be associated with DCM in 60% of patients without structural heart disease, although usually not in the early asymptomatic phase [14–19,21–24,26–32,40,45,53,54,68].

Recommendations for management of diabetic cardiomyopathy

At present, there is no clinically available effective treatment for the LVDD associated with DCM. An investigational agent (ALT-711) that breaks collagen crosslinks formed in the diabetic myocardium under the influence of AGEs eventually may prove to be efficacious and safe in DCM [31]. The ACC/AHA guidelines suggest that the modification of the factors that increase the risk of developing heart failure, such as diabetes, may delay or even prevent its progression [49]. The epidemiologic overlap between type 2 diabetes and heart failure suggests underlying etiologic links and possible opportunities for synergy in therapeutic interventions.

Glycemic control

The UKPDS suggested that intensive glycemic control (target fasting blood glucose <6 mmol/L) with insulin, sulfonylureas, or metformin may reduce the 10-year risk of heart failure compared with conventional therapy (diet alone with supplemental hypoglycemics only for fasting blood glucose >15 mmol/L). In a subgroup of patients inadequately controlled with sulfonylurea therapy alone, the addition of metformin seemed to increase the risk of developing heart failure [69,70]. Intensive therapy was more significantly likely to be associated with hypoglycemic episodes and weight gain than conventional therapy [69].

Thiazolidinediones

Thiazolidinediones are a family of agonists for the nuclear receptor PPARγ. They have ubiquitous actions related to the diffuse nature of their target distribution and the function of nuclear receptor PPARγ in everything from oncogenesis to insulin resistance modulation in the adipocyte. Thiazolidinediones are PPARγ agonists that significantly increase sensitivity to insulin action experimentally and clinically [71,72]. The thiazolidinediones rosiglitazone and pioglitazone offer particularly attractive oral hypoglycemic therapy for possible heart failure risk reduction in individuals with type 2 diabetes and perhaps impaired fasting glucose [71–73].

Thiazolidinediones may have a role in addressing the metabolic abnormalities of diabetic cardiomyopathy by modulating free fatty acids and triglycerides, which results in GLUT4 gene transcription, or thiazolidinediones may effect GLUT4 gene transcription directly. In both cases, insulin-stimulated glucose transport is restored with thiazolidinedione use [72]. PPARγ, in addition to being the target for three insulin-sensitizing agents (the thiazolidinediones), has roles as diverse as adipogenesis, carcinogenesis, and immunomodulation. PPARγ are found predominantly in adipose tissue, but also at lower concentrations in the liver, skeletal muscle, and heart. In the heart, PPARγ are involved in the pathway of carbohydrate metabolism in response to insulin. One group examined Zucker rat (fa/fa) hearts for glucose bioenergetics during exposure to low-flow ischemia and recovery from the same (using glucose uptake evaluated by nuclear magnetic resonance spectroscopy) [72]. The fa/fa hearts during ischemia had a lower glucose uptake and a greater depletion of ATP, and there was an impaired recovery of contractile function during reperfusion. The use of a thiazolidinedione allowed for normalization of insulin-stimulated glucose uptake and prevented the greater loss of ATP and restored recovery of contractile function to that of nondiabetic rat hearts. There was an increased recovery from ischemic insult. It also was noted that there was a concurrent increase in GLUT4 protein expression and a decrease in myocardial free fatty acid and triglyceride levels. This activity also was shown in Wistar rat cardiomyocytes incubated for 20 hours with troglitazone, resulting in a dose-dependent increase in GLUT4 protein expression and improved insulin-stimulated glucose uptake [74]. Liu and coworkers [75] also showed an improvement in insulin-stimulated glucose transport in fa/fa rat cardiomyocytes exposed to a thiazolidinedione (MCC 555) and noted that there seemed to be a twofold increase in phosphatidylinositol 3-kinase activity, connecting and confirming the role of glucose transport and insulin in the activity of thiazolidinediones.

Overall, PPARγ activation improves insulin sensitivity and endothelial function and lowers vascular inflammation and blood pressure, reversing many of the cardiac risk factors associated with diabetes [73]. Clinical application of the knowledge regarding PPARγ agonists has resulted in positive outcomes, increasing expectations that thiazolidinediones might be expected to provide protection from the cardiac effects of hyperglycemia and hyperlipidemia, especially if initiated early in the natural history of the insulin-resistant state [73]. In an experimental model of DCM, treatment with a thiazolidinedione was shown to preserve left ventricular contractility compared with deteriorated myocardial function in untreated animals with the same genetic background [45].

Some concern has been expressed more recently about the risk of worsening established heart failure owing to fluid retention with thiazolidinediones, although no differences were observed between rosiglitazone and placebo in the incidence of new-onset heart failure in clinical trials [76]. Although the AHA and the American Diabetes Association have recommended using thiazolidinediones at lower doses in patients with established asymptomatic left ventricular dysfunction or New York Heart Association (NYHA) class I–II heart failure, and not at all with NYHA class III or IV heart failure patients, clinically important heart failure is rare (<1% with rosiglitazone alone or in combination with sulfonylureas or metformin), and peripheral edema responds well to discontinuation [77]. A more recent study also showed that the use of rosiglitazone for 52 weeks in type 2 diabetic patients with NYHA class I–II heart failure did not adversely alter echocardiographic structure or function, and that fluid-related changes associated with the agent were not due to worsening of congestive heart failure [78]. No significant differences were found in ejection fraction, left ventricular end-diastolic volume, or left ventricular end-systolic volume between the placebo and rosiglitazone groups. Few events of worsening or possible worsening of heart failure were observed; however, more edema and dyspnea were observed in the rosiglitazone-treated patients, but these symptoms were managed by increased use of diuretics. Finally, Masoudi and colleagues [79] in an observational study noted that thiazolidinediones were not associated with increased mortality and may be associated with improved outcomes in older heart failure patients with diabetes.

Neurohumoral inhibition

Treatment for diabetes as stage A heart failure should consist of interventions proven to reduce successfully risk of heart failure–related morbidity and mortality, even in diabetic patients without evidence of LVSD or clinical heart failure [55]. Practice guidelines recommend that the concomitant use of β-blockers and angiotensin-converting enzyme (ACE) inhibitors should be the standard of care for all patients with heart failure secondary to LVSD, regardless of severity or etiology, in the absence of contraindications or intolerance owing to compelling evidence of the cardioprotective benefits shown in clinical trials (Table 2) [54,80,81].

Angiotensin-converting enzyme inhibition

The Heart Outcomes Prevention Evaluation (HOPE) showed the significant benefits of ACE inhibition in patients with documented coronary disease [82]. This study assessed the effects of treatment with the ACE inhibitor ramipril versus placebo in 9297 patients who had evidence of vascular disease or diabetes plus one additional cardiovascular risk factor, but

Table 2
Cardiovascular benefits of angiotensin-converting enzyme inhibition and β blockade

Angiotensin-converting enzyme inhibition	β blockade
Anti-ischemic	Reverses cardiac remodeling
Stimulation of endothelial nitric	Prevents sudden death
oxide production	Anti-ischemic
Reduced myocardial oxygen	Decreases heart rate and blood pressure
consumption	Prolongs diastole (filling coronary arteries)
Antiatherogenic	Decreases myocardial wall stress, which reduces
Lowers systemic vascular resistance	the risk of cardiac rupture owing to decrease
and mean blood pressure	in heart rate and blood pressure
Reduces cardiac afterload and systolic	Antiatherogenic (reduces sheer stress and
wall stress	endothelial dysfunction)
Attenuates remodeling in heart failure	

Data from references [54,80,81].

without left ventricular dysfunction or heart failure. Ramipril treatment reduced the risk of cardiovascular mortality, myocardial infarction, stroke, all-cause mortality, revascularization procedures, cardiac arrest, heart failure, and diabetes-related complications (Fig. 4) [82]. Ramipril treatment reduced the risk of new-onset heart failure by 23%.

A substudy, MICRO-HOPE, examined whether ramipril could lower the risks of cardiovascular and renal disease in 3577 patients with diabetes [83]. Ramipril reduced the risk of total mortality by 24%, myocardial infarction by 22%, stroke by 33%, cardiovascular death by 37%, and revascularization by 17%. These results from HOPE and MICRO-HOPE provide convincing evidence that ACE inhibitors can lower the risk of new-onset heart failure in patients with diabetes. An analysis of major clinical trials shows that diabetic patients with heart failure benefit from therapy with ACE inhibitors to a similar degree as their nondiabetic counterparts (Table 3) [84].

β Blockade

The UKPDS showed that patients who were assigned to tight blood pressure control with ACE inhibitors and β-blockers experienced a remarkable 56% heart failure risk reduction with either therapy [85]. In patients with established heart failure, β-blockers have produced substantial mortality reductions. Post-hoc analyses and meta-analyses have questioned whether heart failure patients with diabetes benefit as much from β-blocker therapy as patients without diabetes. These analyses have combined outcomes from the subpopulation of patients with diabetes included in the large β-blocker heart failure trials and have concluded that although β-blockers reduce mortality in diabetic heart failure patients, the reduction may not be as great as that seen in the nondiabetic subject [84,86–88]. The effects of β-blockers on diabetic and nondiabetic subjects are summarized in Table 4 [89–93].

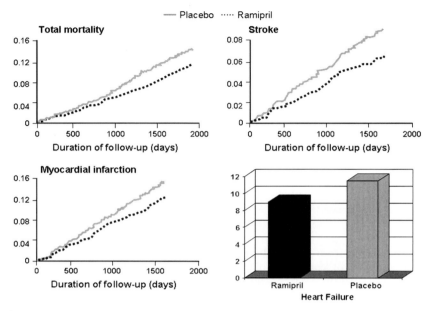

Fig. 4. Cardiovascular events in diabetic patients who participated in the Heart Outcomes Prevention Evaluation (HOPE) study. Relative risk reduction with ramipril therapy compared with placebo was 24% for total mortality, 33% for stroke, and 22% for myocardial infarction. (*Adapted from* Yusuf S, Sleight P, Pogue J, et al. Effects of an angiotensin-converting-enzyme inhibitor, ramipril, on cardiovascular events in high-risk patients. The Heart Outcomes Prevention Evaluation Study Investigators [published errata appear in N Engl J Med 2000 Mar 9;342(10):748 and 2000 May 4;342(18):1376]. N Engl J Med 2000;342:145–53; with permission.)

In the Metoprolol Controlled-Release Randomized Intervention Trial in Heart Failure (MERIT-HF), metoprolol succinate proved statistically beneficial in the entire heart failure population; however, there was a statistically nonsignificant trend toward decreased all-cause mortality in metoprolol-treated diabetic patients [94]. Likewise, in the Cardiac Insufficiency Bisoprolol Study II (CIBIS-II), which studied the effects of bisoprolol in heart failure patients, there was a statistically nonsignificant trend toward reduced mortality in bisoprolol-treated diabetic patients [95].

The Carvedilol Prospective Randomized Cumulative Survival Study (COPERNICUS) enrolled more than 2200 patients with severe heart failure symptoms at rest or on minimal exertion (NYHA class IV heart failure) and an ejection fraction of less than 25%; carvedilol use resulted in a 35% reduction in all-cause mortality in all patients [92]. The effect of β blockade on all-cause mortality in heart failure by diabetic status for three major heart failure trials is shown in Fig. 5 [94,96,97]. In COPERNICUS, the relative risk reduction in all-cause mortality was exactly the same for diabetic and nondiabetic patients treated with carvedilol: 35% [98]. In addition, in the US Carvedilol

Table 3
Effect of angiotensin-converting enzyme inhibitors on mortality in diabetic and nondiabetic heart failure patients

Study	Patients (n)			Relative risk (95% CI)		
	Total	Nondiabetic	Diabetic	Nondiabetic	Diabetic	Ratio
CONSENSUS	253	197	56	0.64 (0.46, 0.88)	1.06 (0.65, 1.74)	1.67 (0.93, 3.01)
SAVE	2231	1739	492	0.82 (0.68, 0.99)	0.89 (0.68, 1.16)	1.09 (0.79, 1.50)
SMILE	1556	1253	303	0.79 (0.54, 1.15)	0.44 (0.22, 0.87)	0.56 (0.25, 1.22)
SOLVD-Prevention	4228	3581	647	0.97 (0.83, 1.15)	0.75 (0.55, 1.02)	0.77 (0.54, 1.09)
SOLVD-Treatment	2569	1906	663	0.84 (0.74, 0.95)	1.01 (0.85, 1.21)	1.21 (0.97, 1.50)
TRACE	1749	1512	237	0.85 (0.74, 0.97)	0.73 (0.57, 0.94)	0.87 (0.65, 1.15)
Random effects pooled estimate		10,188	2398	0.85 (0.78, 0.92)	0.84 (0.70, 1.00)	1.00 (0.80, 1.25)

Abbreviations: CONSENSUS, Cooperative North Scandinavian Enalapril Survival Study; SAVE, Survival and Ventricular Enlargement; SMILE, Survival of Myocardial Infarction Long-term Evaluation; SOLVD, Studies of Left Ventricular Dysfunction; TRACE, Trandolapril Cardiac Evaluation.
From Shekelle PG, Rich MW, Morton SC, et al. Efficacy of angiotensin-converting enzyme inhibitors and beta-blockers in the management of left ventricular systolic dysfunction according to race, gender and diabetic status: a meta-analysis of major clinical trials. J Am Coll Cardiol 2003;41:1529–38.

Table 4
Effect of β-blockers on mortality in diabetic and nondiabetic heart failure patients

Study	Diabetic patients (%)	β-blocker	Heart failure severity	Target dosage	Mortality decrease: all patients	Mortality decrease: diabetic patients
US Carvedilol Program	29	Carvedilol	Mild/moderate/severe	6.25–25 mg bid*	65%[†] (P < .001)	63% (8%, 85%)
CIBIS-II	12	Bisoprolol[‡]	Moderate/severe	10 mg qd	34% (P < .0001)	19% P = NS
MERIT-HF	25	Metoprolol succinate	Mild/moderate	200 mg qd	34% (P = .0062)	18% P = NS
COPERNICUS	26	Carvedilol	Severe	25 mg bid	35% (P = .0014)	32% P = NS
ANZ	19	Carvedilol	Mild/moderate	25 mg bid	24%[†] (P = NS)	56% P = NS

Abbreviations: ANZ, Australia/New Zealand Heart Failure Trial; CIBIS-II, Cardiac Insufficiency Bisoprolol Study II; COPERNICUS, Carvedilol Prospective Randomized Cumulative Survival; MERIT-HF, Metoprolol CR/XL Randomised Intervention Trial in Congestive Heart Failure.

* 50 mg bid if patient weighed >85 kg.
[†] Not a planned end point.
[‡] Heart failure is not an approved indication.
Data from references [89–93].

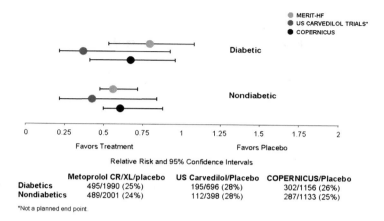

Fig. 5. Effect of β blockade on all-cause mortality in heart failure by diabetic status. COPER-NICUS, Carvedilol Prospective Randomized Cumulative Survival; MERIT-HF, Metoprolol Controlled-Release Randomized Intervention Trial in Heart Failure. (*Data from* references [87,89,90].)

Trials, carvedilol treatment was associated with a significant reduction in all-cause mortality in diabetic patients with heart failure [97].

Diabetic heart failure patients are less likely to receive β-blockers in part because of their adverse effects on glycemic control and blood lipids [98]. The Glycemic Effects in Diabetes Mellitus: Carvedilol-Metoprolol Comparison in Hypertensives (GEMINI) study reported that blood pressure–lowering therapy with the β-blocker carvedilol did not adversely affect glycemic control in diabetic patients, in contrast to metoprolol tartrate. Although carvedilol had a neutral effect on mean hemoglobin A_{1c} levels, metoprolol tartrate significantly increased mean hemoglobin A_{1c} by 0.15%. Although insulin resistance nonsignificantly increased with metoprolol tartrate, it significantly decreased with carvedilol, for a mean difference of 7.2% between the treatment groups [99]. The neutral or beneficial metabolic effects of carvedilol in the diabetic heart failure patient, coupled with the proven mortality and morbidity benefits of neurohormonal blockade in all patients with heart failure, support the use of this β-blocker in conjunction with an ACE inhibitor as standard therapy for all diabetic patients with heart failure.

Aldosterone blockade

Aldosterone promotes myocardial and vascular fibrosis and has numerous other deleterious effects in heart failure. Because aldosterone production is incompletely suppressed by ACE inhibitor therapy, aldosterone blockade in patients with heart failure has been thought to provide additional benefits. One study of aldosterone blockade, the Eplerenone Post–Acute Myocardial

Infarction Heart Failure Efficacy and Survival Study (EPHESUS), investigated the subgroup of diabetic patients in the trial: All-cause mortality was reduced by 15% in all patients treated with eplerenone. Patients with diabetes ($n = 2122$) also benefited from aldosterone blockade, and there was no significant heterogeneity with respect to mortality benefit between diabetic and nondiabetic patients [100].

Summary

Patients with diabetes are at an elevated risk for heart failure, and comorbid heart failure confers an increased risk of morbidity and mortality. DCM is a distinctive syndrome that confers high risk of morbidity and mortality. Clinical trials have shown that combined neurohormonal blockade with the use of ACE inhibitors, aldosterone antagonists, and β-blockers can decrease the risk for cardiovascular events and mortality in patients with heart failure and diabetes. Every effort should be made to diagnose patients with DCM and to apply proven lifesaving therapies in all heart failure patients, including diabetics, in the absence of contraindications or intolerance.

References

[1] Richardson P, McKenna W, Bristow M, et al. Report of the 1995 World Health Organization/International Society and Federation of Cardiology Task Force on the Definition and Classification of cardiomyopathies. Circulation 1996;93:841–2.

[2] Narula J, Virmani R, Ballester M, et al. Heart failure: pathogenesis and treatment. New York: Isis Medical Media/Taylor & Francis; 2002.

[3] Haffner SM, Lehto S, Ronnemaa T, et al. Mortality from coronary heart disease in subjects with type 2 diabetes and in nondiabetic subjects with and without prior myocardial infarction. N Engl J Med 1998;339:229–34.

[4] Kannel WB, McGee DL. Diabetes and cardiovascular disease: the Framingham study. JAMA 1979;241:2035–8.

[5] Schannwell CM, Schneppenheim M, Perings S, et al. Left ventricular diastolic dysfunction as an early manifestation of diabetic cardiomyopathy. Cardiology 2002;98:33–9.

[6] Poirier P, Bogaty P, Garneau C, et al. Diastolic dysfunction in normotensive men with well-controlled type 2 diabetes: importance of maneuvers in echocardiographic screening for preclinical diabetic cardiomyopathy. Diabetes Care 2001;24:5–10.

[7] Valle R, Bagolin E, Canali C, et al. The BNP assay does not identify mild left ventricular diastolic dysfunction in asymptomatic diabetic patients. Eur J Echocardiogr 2006;7:40–4.

[8] Bell DSH. Diabetic cardiomyopathy: a unique entity or a complication of coronary artery disease? Diabetes Care 1995;18:708–14.

[9] Devereux RB, Roman MJ, Paranicas M, et al. Impact of diabetes on cardiac structure and function: the strong heart study. Circulation 2000;101:2271–6.

[10] Fang ZY, Yuda S, Anderson V, et al. Echocardiographic detection of early diabetic myocardial disease. J Am Coll Cardiol 2003;41:611–7.

[11] Vinereanu D, Nicolaides E, Tweddel AC, et al. Subclinical left ventricular dysfunction in asymptomatic patients with type II diabetes mellitus, related to serum lipids and glycated haemoglobin. Clin Sci (Lond) 2003;105:591–9.

[12] Ungar I, Gilbert M, Siegel A, et al. Studies on myocardial metabolism: IV. myocardial metabolism in diabetes. Am J Med 1955;18:385–96.

[13] Howard BV, Rodriguez BL, Bennett PH, et al. Prevention Conference VI: diabetes and cardiovascular disease. Writing Group I: epidemiology. Circulation 2002;105:e132–7.

[14] Giles TD, Sander GE. Diabetes mellitus and heart failure: basic mechanisms, clinical features, and therapeutic considerations. Cardiol Clin 2004;22:553–68.

[15] Goldstein BJ. Insulin resistance as the core defect in type 2 diabetes mellitus. Am J Cardiol 2002;90:3G–10G.

[16] Festa A, D'Agostino R Jr, Hales CN, et al. Heart rate in relation to insulin sensitivity and insulin secretion in nondiabetic subjects. Diabetes Care 2000;23:624–8.

[17] Gillum RF, Makuc DM, Feldman JJ. Pulse rate, coronary heart disease, and death: the NHANES I Epidemiologic Follow-up Study. Am Heart J 1991;121:172–7.

[18] Kannel WB, Kannel C, Paffenbarger RS Jr, et al. Heart rate and cardiovascular mortality: the Framingham Study. Am Heart J 1987;113:1489–94.

[19] Taegtmeyer H, McNulty P, Young ME. Adaptation and maladaptation of the heart in diabetes: Part I. general concepts. Circulation 2002;105:1727–33.

[20] Malmberg K, Ryden L, Hamsten A, et al. Effects of insulin treatment on cause-specific one-year mortality and morbidity in diabetic patients with acute myocardial infarction. DIGAMI Study Group. Diabetes Insulin-Glucose in Acute Myocardial Infarction. Eur Heart J 1996;17:1337–44.

[21] Darnell J, Lodish H, Baltimore D. Cellular genetics: formation of ATP by glycolysis and oxidative phosphorylation. In: Molecular cell biology. New York: WH Freeman Company/Scientific American Books; 1990. p. 743–5.

[22] McNulty PH, Louard RJ, Deckelbaum LI, et al. Hyperinsulinemia inhibits myocardial protein degradation in patients with cardiovascular disease and insulin resistance. Circulation 1995;92:2151–6.

[23] Egan BM. Insulin resistance and the sympathetic nervous system. Curr Hypertens Rep 2003;5:247–54.

[24] Packer M. Beta-adrenergic blockade in chronic heart failure: principles, progress, and practice. Prog Cardiovasc Dis 1998;41:39–52.

[25] Ye G, Donthi RV, Metrevel NS, et al. Cardiomyocyte dysfunction in models of type 1 and type 2 diabetes. Cardiovasc Toxicol 2005;5:285–92.

[26] Bell DS. Diabetic cardiomyopathy. Diabetes Care 2003;26:2949–51.

[27] Norton GR, Candy G, Woodiwiss AJ. Aminoguanidine prevents the decreased myocardial compliance produced by streptozotocin-induced diabetes mellitus in rats. Circulation 1996; 93:1905–12.

[28] Avendano GF, Agarwal RK, Bashey RI, et al. Effects of glucose intolerance on myocardial function and collagen-linked glycation. Diabetes 1999;48:1443–7.

[29] Liu J, Masurekar MR, Vatner DE, et al. Glycation end-product cross-link breaker reduces collagen and improves cardiac function in aging diabetic heart. Am J Physiol Heart Circ Physiol 2003;285:H2587–91.

[30] Brownlee M, Cerami A, Vlassara H. Advanced glycosylation end products in tissue and the biochemical basis of diabetic complications. N Engl J Med 1988;318:1315–21.

[31] Candido R, Forbes JM, Thomas MC, et al. A breaker of advanced glycation end products attenuates diabetes-induced myocardial structural changes. Circ Res 2003;92: 785–92.

[32] Yu Y, Ohmori K, Kondo I, et al. Correlation of functional and structural alterations of the coronary arterioles during development of type II diabetes mellitus in rats. Cardiovasc Res 2002;56:303–11.

[33] Singal PK, Bello-Klein A, Farahmand F, et al. Oxidative stress and functional deficit in diabetic cardiomyopathy. Adv Exp Med Biol 2001;498:213–20.

[34] Liang Q, Carlson EC, Donthi RV, et al. Overexpression of metallothionein reduces diabetic cardiomyopathy. Diabetes 2002;51:174–81.

[35] Liu X, Wang J, Takeda N, et al. Changes in cardiac protein kinase C activities and isozymes in streptozotocin-induced diabetes. Am J Physiol 1999;277:E798–804.

[36] Abe T, Ohga Y, Tabayashi N, et al. Left ventricular diastolic dysfunction in type 2 diabetes mellitus model rats. Am J Physiol Heart Circ Physiol 2002;282:H138–48.

[37] Golfman L, Dixon IM, Takeda N, et al. Cardiac sarcolemmal Na(+)-Ca2+ exchange and Na(+)-K+ ATPase activities and gene expression in alloxan-induced diabetes in rats. Mol Cell Biochem 1998;188:91–101.

[38] Nakajima T, Iwasawa K, Oonuma H, et al. Troglitazone inhibits voltage-dependent calcium currents in guinea pig cardiac myocytes. Circulation 1999;99:2942–50.

[39] Rozanski GJ, Xu Z. A metabolic mechanism for cardiac K+ channel remodelling. Clin Exp Pharmacol Physiol 2002;29:132–7.

[40] Young ME, McNulty P, Taegtmeyer H. Adaptation and maladaptation of the heart in diabetes: Part II. potential mechanisms. Circulation 2002;105:1861–70.

[41] Guerre-Millo M, Rovault C, Poulain P, et al. PPAR-alpha-null mice are protected from high-fat diet-induced insulin resistance. Diabetes 2001;50:2809–14.

[42] Roduit R, Morin J, Masse F, et al. Glucose down-regulates the expression of the peroxisome proliferator-activated receptor alpha gene in the pancreatic beta -cell. J Biol Chem 2000;275:35799–806.

[43] Finck BN, Lehman JJ, Leone TC, et al. The cardiac phenotype induced by PPARalpha overexpression mimics that caused by diabetes mellitus. J Clin Invest 2002;109:121–30.

[44] Yagyu H, Chen G, Yokoyuma M, et al. Lipoprotein lipase (LpL) on the surface of cardiomyocytes increases lipid uptake and produces a cardiomyopathy. J Clin Invest 2003;111:419–26.

[45] Zhou YT, Grayburn P, Karim A, et al. Lipotoxic heart disease in obese rats: implications for human obesity. Proc Natl Acad Sci U S A 2000;97:1784–9.

[46] Rubler S, Dlugash J, Yuceoglu YZ, et al. New type of cardiomyopathy associated with diabetic glomerulosclerosis. Am J Cardiol 1972;30:595–602.

[47] Sima A, Popov D, Starodub O, et al. Pathobiology of the heart in experimental diabetes: immunolocalization of lipoproteins, immunoglobulin G, and advanced glycation endproducts proteins in diabetic and/or hyperlipidemic hamster. Lab Invest 1997;77:3–18.

[48] Regan TJ, Lyons MM, Ahmed SS, et al. Evidence for cardiomyopathy in familial diabetes mellitus. J Clin Invest 1977;60:884–99.

[49] Moir S, Hanekom L, Fang ZY, et al. The relationship between myocardial perfusion and dysfunction in diabetic cardiomyopathy: a study of quantitative contrast echocardiography and strain rate imaging. Heart 2006.

[50] Scognamiglio R, Casara D, Avogaro A. Myocardial dysfunction and adrenergic innervation in patients with type 1 diabetes mellitus. Diabetes Nutr Metab 2000;13:346–9.

[51] Kahn JK, Zola B, Juni JE, et al. Radionuclide assessment of left ventricular diastolic filling in diabetes mellitus with and without cardiac autonomic neuropathy. J Am Coll Cardiol 1986;7:1303–9.

[52] Monteagudo PT, Moises VA, Kohlmann O Jr, et al. Influence of autonomic neuropathy upon left ventricular dysfunction in insulin-dependent diabetic patients. Clin Cardiol 2000;23:371–5.

[53] Diamant M, Lamb HJ, Groeneveld Y, et al. Diastolic dysfunction is associated with altered myocardial metabolism inasymptomatic normotensive patientswith well-controlled type 2 diabetes mellitus. J Am Coll Cardiol 2003;42:328–35.

[54] Edwin JK, Garrison JC. Renin and angiotensin. In: Hardman JG, Limbird LE, Molinoff PB, et al, editors. Goodman and Gilman's the pharmacological basis of therapeutics. New York: McGraw-Hill; 1996. p. 734–58.

[55] Hunt SA, Baker DW, Chin MH, et al. ACC/AHA guidelines for the evaluation and management of chronic heart failure in the adult: executive summary. A report of the American College of Cardiology/American Heart Association Task Force on Practice Guidelines (Committee to revise the 1995 Guidelines for the Evaluation and Management of Heart Failure). J Am Coll Cardiol 2001;38:2101–13.

[56] Fonarow GC, Adams K, Strausser BP. ADHERE (Acute Decompensated Heart Failure National Registry): rationale, design, and subject population. J Card Fail 2002;8:S49.

[57] Nichols GA, Hillier TA, Erbey JR, et al. Congestive heart failure in type 2 diabetes: prevalence, incidence, and risk factors. Diabetes Care 2001;24:1614–9.

[58] Chae CU, Glynn RJ, Manson JE, et al. Diabetes predicts congestive heart failure risk in the elderly. Circulation 1998;98(Suppl 1):I-658.

[59] Iribarren C, Karter AJ, Go AS, et al. Glycemic control and heart failure among adult patients with diabetes. Circulation 2001;103:2668–73.

[60] Bertoni AG, Tsai A, Kasper EK, et al. Diabetes and idiopathic cardiomyopathy: a nationwide case-control study. Diabetes Care 2003;26:2791–5.

[61] Stratton IM, Adler AI, Neil HA, et al. Association of glycaemia with macrovascular and microvascular complications of type 2 diabetes (UKPDS 35): prospective observational study. BMJ 2000;321:405–12.

[62] Shehadeh A, Regan TJ. Cardiac consequences of diabetes mellitus. Clin Cardiol 1995;18: 301–5.

[63] Raev DC. Which left ventricular function is impaired earlier in the evolution of diabetic cardiomyopathy? An echocardiographic study of young type I diabetic patients. Diabetes Care 1994;17:633–9.

[64] Arnlov J, Lind L, Zethelius B, et al. Several factors associated with the insulin resistance syndrome are predictors of left ventricular systolic dysfunction in a male population after 20 years of follow-up. Am Heart J 2001;142:720–4.

[65] Fang ZY, Najos-Valencia O, Leano R, et al. Patients with early diabetic heart disease demonstrate a normal myocardial response to dobutamine. J Am Coll Cardiol 2003; 42:446–53.

[66] Redfield MM, Jacobsen SJ, Burnett JC Jr, et al. Burden of systolic and diastolic ventricular dysfunction in the community: appreciating the scope of the heart failure epidemic. JAMA 2003;289:194–202.

[67] Shindler DM, Kostis JB, Yusuf S, et al. Diabetes mellitus, a predictor of morbidity and mortality in the Studies of Left Ventricular Dysfunction (SOLVD) Trials and Registry. Am J Cardiol 1996;77:1017–20.

[68] Casis O, Echevarria E. Diabetic cardiomyopathy: electromechanical cellular alterations. Curr Vasc Pharmacol 2004;2:237–48.

[69] UK Prospective Diabetes Study (UKPDS) Group. Intensive blood-glucose control with sulphonylureas or insulin compared with conventional treatment and risk of complications in patients with type 2 diabetes (UKPDS 33). Lancet 1998;352:837–53.

[70] UKPD Study Group. Effect of intensive blood-glucose control with metformin on complications in overweight patients with type 2 diabetes (UKPDS 34). UK Prospective Diabetes Study (UKPDS) Group. Lancet 1998;352:854–65.

[71] Saltiel AR, Olefsky JM. Thiazolidinediones in the treatment of insulin resistance and type II diabetes. Diabetes 1996;45:1661–9.

[72] Sidell RJ, Cole MA, Draper NJ, et al. Thiazolidinedione treatment normalizes insulin resistance and ischemic injury in the Zucker fatty rat heart. Diabetes 2002;51:1110–7.

[73] Wang CH, Weisel RD, Liu PP, et al. Glitazones and heart failure: critical appraisal for the clinician. Circulation 2003;107:1350–4.

[74] Bahr M, Spelleken M, Bock M, et al. Acute and chronic effects of troglitazone (CS-045) on isolated rat ventricular cardiomyocytes. Diabetologia 1996;39:766–74.

[75] Liu LS, Tanaka H, Ishii S, et al. The new antidiabetic drug MCC-555 acutely sensitizes insulin signaling in isolated cardiomyocytes. Endocrinology 1998;139:4531–9.

[76] Hollenberg NK. Considerations for management of fluid dynamic issues associated with thiazolidinediones. Am J Med 2003;115(Suppl 8A):111S–5S.

[77] Nesto RW, Bell D, Bonow RO, et al. Thiazolidinedione use, fluid retention, and congestive heart failure: a consensus statement from the American Heart Association and American Diabetes Association. Circulation 2003;108:2941–8.

[78] Wilding J, Dargie H, Hildebrandt P, et al. Rosiglitazone (RSG) administered to patients with type 2 diabetes (T2DM) and class I/II congestive heart failure (CHF) does not adversely affect echocardiographic structure or function parameters. American Diabetes Association; 2005. Available at: http://scientificsession.diabetes.org. Accessed August 1, 2006.

[79] Masoudi FA, Inzucchi SE, Wang Y, et al. Thiazolidinediones, metformin, and outcomes in older patients with diabetes and heart failure: an observational study. Circulation 2005;111: 583–90.

[80] Tse WY, Kendall M. Is there a role for beta-blockers in hypertensive diabetic patients? Diabet Med 1994;11:137–44.

[81] Pepine CJ. Potential role of angiotensin-converting enzyme inhibition in myocardial ischemia and current clinical trials. Clin Cardiol 1997;20:II-58–64.

[82] Yusuf S, Sleight P, Pogue J, et al. Effects of an angiotensin-converting-enzyme inhibitor, ramipril, on cardiovascular events in high-risk patients. The Heart Outcomes Prevention Evaluation Study Investigators [published errata appear in N Engl J Med 2000 Mar 9;342(10):748 and 2000 May 4;342(18):1376]. N Engl J Med 2000;342:145–53.

[83] Heart Outcomes Prevention Evaluation Study investigators. Effects of ramipril on cardiovascular and microvascular outcomes in people with diabetes mellitus: results of the HOPE study and MICRO-HOPE substudy. Lancet 2000;355:253–9.

[84] Shekelle PG, Rich MW, Morton SC, et al. Efficacy of angiotensin-converting enzyme inhibitors and beta-blockers in the management of left ventricular systolic dysfunction according to race, gender, and diabetic status: a meta-analysis of major clinical trials. J Am Coll Cardiol 2003;41:1529–38.

[85] UKPD Study Group. Tight blood pressure control and risk of macrovascular and microvascular complications in type 2 diabetes: UKPDS 38. UK Prospective Diabetes Study Group. BMJ 1998;317:703–13.

[86] Bobbio M, Ferrua S, Opasich C, et al. Survival and hospitalization in heart failure patients with or without diabetes treated with beta-blockers. J Card Fail 2003;9:192–202.

[87] Haas SJ, Vos T, Gilbert RE, et al. Are beta-blockers as efficacious in patients with diabetes mellitus as in patients without diabetes mellitus who have chronic heart failure? A meta-analysis of large-scale clinical trials. Am Heart J 2003;146:848–53.

[88] Deedwania PC, Giles TD, Klibaner M, et al. Efficacy, safety and tolerability of metoprolol CR/XL in patients with diabetes and chronic heart failure: experiences from MERIT-HF. Am Heart J 2005;149:159–67.

[89] Packer M, Bristow MR, Cohn JN, et al. The effect of carvedilol on morbidity and mortality in patients with chronic heart failure. U.S. Carvedilol Heart Failure Study Group. N Engl J Med 1996;334:1349–55.

[90] CIBIS-II investigators. The Cardiac Insufficiency Bisoprolol Study II (CIBIS-II): a randomised trial. Lancet 1999;353:9–13.

[91] MERIT-HF investigators. Effect of metoprolol CR/XL in chronic heart failure: Metoprolol CR/XL Randomised Intervention Trial in Congestive Heart Failure (MERIT-HF). Lancet 1999;353:2001–7.

[92] Packer M, Coats AJS, Fowler MB, et al. Effect of carvedilol on survival in severe chronic heart failure. N Engl J Med 2001;344:1651–8.

[93] Australia/New Zealand Heart Failure Research Collaborative Group. Randomised, placebo-controlled trial of carvedilol in patients with congestive heart failure due to ischaemic heart disease. Australia/New Zealand Heart Failure Research Collaborative Group. Lancet 1997;349:375–80.

[94] Wedel H, DeMets D, Deedwania P, et al. Challenges of subgroup analyses in multinational clinical trials: experiences from the MERIT-HF trial. Am Heart J 2001;142:502–11.

[95] Erdmann E, Lechat P, Verkenne P, et al. Results from post-hoc analyses of the CIBIS II trial: effect of bisoprolol in high-risk patient groups with chronic heart failure. Eur J Heart Fail 2001;3:469–79.

[96] Mohacsi P, Fowler MB, Krum H, et al. Should physicians avoid the use of beta-blockers in patients with heart failure who have diabetes? Results of the COPERNICUS study. Presented at the American Heart Association 74th Annual Scientific Session. Anaheim (CA), November 14, 2001 [abstract 3551]. Circulation 2001;104(Suppl II):II-754.

[97] Bristow MR. Effect of carvedilol on LV function and mortality in diabetic vs non-diabetic patients with ischemic or nonischemic dilated cardiomyopathy. Presented at the 69th Scientific Sessions, New Orleans Convention Center. New Orleans, November 10-13, 1996. Circulation 1996;84:I-644.

[98] Lithell HO. Effect of antihypertensive drugs on insulin, glucose, and lipid metabolism. Diabetes Care 1991;14:203–9.

[99] Bakris GL, Fonseca V, Katholi RE, et al. Metabolic effects of carvedilol vs metoprolol in patients with type 2 diabetes mellitus and hypertension: a randomized controlled trial. JAMA 2004;292:2227–36.

[100] Pitt B, Remme W, Zannad F, et al. Eplerenone, a selective aldosterone blocker, in patients with left ventricular dysfunction after myocardial infarction. N Engl J Med 2003;348: 1309–21.

ELSEVIER
SAUNDERS

Endocrinol Metab Clin N Am
35 (2006) 601–610

ENDOCRINOLOGY
AND METABOLISM
CLINICS
OF NORTH AMERICA

Alterations in Ion Channel Physiology in Diabetic Cardiomyopathy

David A. Cesario, MD, PhD, Ramandeep Brar, MD,
Kalyanam Shivkumar, MD, PhD*

*UCLA Cardiac Arrhythmia Center, Division of Cardiology, Department of Medicine,
David Geffen School of Medicine at UCLA, 47-123 CHS,
10833 Le Conte Avenue, Los Angeles, CA 90095, USA*

Diabetes mellitus is one of the most common chronic diseases worldwide. Cardiovascular complications are the leading causes of morbidity and mortality among diabetic patients. Diabetes mellitus is associated with cardiovascular disease related to coronary artery atherosclerosis, autonomic neuropathy, macroangiopathy, and microcirculatory disorders [1]. Diabetes mellitus has been shown to induce multiple abnormal pathologic findings, including cell hypertrophy, intracardiac lipid deposition, neuropathy, interstitial fibrosis, and loss of cardiac myocytes through cell lysis and apoptosis. Diabetes mellitus induces changes in the heart that affect the structure of the plasma membrane, mitochondria, and sarcoplasmic reticulum of cardiac myocytes and changes in the morphology of the cardiac interstitium [2].

This article focuses on a subgroup of diabetic patients with a specific cardiac complication of the disease—diabetic cardiomyopathy. First, some general background on diabetic cardiomyopathy and ion channels is given. Next the authors focus on how diabetic cardiomyopathy alters calcium homeostasis in cardiac myocytes and highlight the specific alterations in ion channel function that are characteristic of this type of cardiomyopathy. Finally, the importance of the renin-angiotensin system in diabetic cardiomyopathy is reviewed.

Diabetic cardiomyopathy

Diabetic cardiomyopathy is a disease state specific to diabetic patients that occurs in the absence of many traditional cardiac risk factors. The

---

This article was supported by grants from the American Heart Association and the National Heart Lung and Blood Institute R01 HL084261 (K. Shivkumar).
* Corresponding author.
E-mail address: kshivkumar@mednet.ucla.edu (K. Shivkumar).

doi:10.1016/j.ecl.2006.05.002

syndrome of diabetic cardiomyopathy includes cardiomegaly, left ventricular dysfunction, electrical remodeling of the ventricle, and congestive heart
failure symptoms [3–6]. The electrophysiologic changes resulting from diabetic cardiomyopathy likely contribute to the increased incidence of cardiac
arrhythmias and sudden death seen in this patient population and have been
associated with changes in the surface electrocardiogram, including T wave
abnormalities and QT prolongation [7].

The etiology of diabetic cardiomyopathy is complex, and several factors
have been implicated in the pathogenesis of this disease, including (1) variations in cardiac metabolism, (2) decreased vascular sensitivity and abnormal reactivity to various ligands, (3) increased ventricular wall stiffness
with associated perivascular thickening of the basement membrane and interstitial accumulation of glycoprotein and insoluble collagen, and (4) abnormalities of various ion channels that control ionic homeostasis across
the cell membrane. Intracellular calcium abnormalities have been well characterized in diabetic cardiomyopathy patients [5,8]. Diabetic cardiomyopathy has been linked to multiple metabolic disturbances and an increase in
reactive oxygen species that together result in depressed myocyte function
[9,10]. Hyperglycemia is a known cause of reactive oxygen species and reactive nitrogen species release [11]. The release of reactive oxygen and nitrogen
species leads to abnormal gene expression, abnormal signal transduction,
and ultimately apoptosis of cardiac myocytes. Hyperglycemia also can induce programmed cell death via p53 and activation of the cytochrome-c–
activated caspase-3 pathway [11,12]. In diabetic hearts, oxidative stress
and impaired calcium transport contribute to cardiac myocyte loss and abnormalities in excitation contraction coupling.

Ion channels

Ion channels are a diverse group of pore-forming proteins that transverse
the cell membrane and allow the selective passage of ions across this lipid
barrier. Ion channels are the major transducers of intercellular physiologic
signals and are particularly important in the heart, where they play a vital
role in every heartbeat [13]. The cardiac action potential depends on the coordinated actions of numerous different ion channels in the sacrolemma.
The organized cardiac activation sequence, progressing from the sinoatrial
node to the ventricle, is directly mediated by intercellular ion channels (con-
nexons) between adjacent myocytes. Changes in membrane potential and
the flow of ions through sarcolemmal ion channels regulate another group
of ion channels located on intracellular organelles. These subcellular ion
channels regulate contractile force by controlling calcium release from inter-
nal stores and determine energy production by the cellular metabolic
machinery. Intracellular calcium is the central regulator of cardiac contrac-
tililty. Alterations in myocyte calcium regulation play an important role in
the mechanical dysfunction and arrhythmogenesis seen in congestive heart

failure [14,15]. There is a growing body of evidence that intracellular calcium metabolism is impaired in diabetes mellitus and more specifically in the cardiac myocytes of patients with diabetic cardiomyopathy.

Importance of animal models in studying diabetic cardiomyopathy

Animal models have been particularly useful in defining abnormalities in calcium homeostasis in diabetes. Streptozocin is one agent that can induce diabetes in rats through its selective cytotoxic action on pancreatic β cells [8]. Rats treated with streptozocin develop depressed left ventricular contractility, decreased ventricular compliance, and blunted inotropic and chronotropic responses to certain medications in isolated myocardial preparations [4,16,17]. Additionally, alterations in contractile proteins have been described in streptozocin-induced diabetic rats [18,19]. The hearts of streptozocin-induced diabetic rats develop a neuropathy associated with a reduction in axon number and ganglia with swollen mitochondria and abnormal neurofilaments and neurotubules [2,20]. Diabetic rats have parasympathetic nervous system abnormalities, similar to the neuropathy seen in humans with diabetes [21]. Streptozocin-induced diabetic rats do not develop atherosclerosis, and the cardiac contractile and metabolic abnormalities likely reflect a change in myocardial cell function [22]. These properties make the streptozocin-induced diabetic rat a useful model to study the pathogenesis of diabetic cardiomyopathy.

Importance of calcium homeostasis in normal cardiac function

The movement of calcium is an important determinant of cardiac electromechanical events, energy metabolism, and contractile function. The maintenance of intracellular free calcium concentration requires the coordinated control of multiple organelles. In the ventricular myocyte, calcium moves across the sarcolemma, sarcoplasmic reticulum, and mitochondrial membranes through various ion channels and ion transporters, including L-type calcium channels, sodium-calcium exchangers, calcium-ATPases, calcium release channels, and calcium binding proteins. During myocardial excitation, extracellular calcium moves into cardiac myocytes through activated calcium channels and reverse sodium-calcium exchange [23,24]. This influx of calcium results in a release of calcium from the sarcoplasmic reticulum, via the ryanodine receptors, in a process known as calcium-induced calcium release [25]. This sudden increase in cytosolic free calcium results in calcium binding to multiple buffers, including the thin filament protein cardiac troponin C. When calcium binds troponin C, it results in myofilament activation ultimately leading to contraction [26]. For relaxation and diastolic filling to occur, cytosolic calcium concentration must decline, so it dissociates from troponin C resulting in a termination of contraction. Four different transporters remove calcium from the cytosol: (1) the sarcoplasmic reticulum calcium-ATPase, (2) sarcolemmal sodium-calcium exchanger, (3) sarcolemmal calcium-ATPase, and (4) the mitochondrial calcium uniporter [26].

Altered cardiac calcium homeostasis in diabetes

During chronic diabetes, cardiac intracellular calcium homeostasis is altered. Some evidence suggests that this altered calcium homeostasis is the result of impaired sarcoplasmic reticulum function [27]. In diabetic hearts, the sarcolemmal calcium pump and sodium-calcium exchanger activity are decreased, and abnormalities in mitochondrial calcium have been reported [28–30]. Isolated cardiac myocytes from diabetic rats display overall impaired contraction, decreased cell shortening, and a lower relaxation velocity than control cells [31,32]. It originally was thought that these abnormalities in cardiac myocyte contractile function were due to calcium overload [33,34]. Subsequent data suggest, however, that basal cytosolic calcium levels are not altered in diabetic cardiac myocytes [35,36]. These findings led to the hypothesis that abnormalities in cytosolic calcium transients, rather than altered basal calcium levels, were likely the cause of depressed myocyte function.

Specific ion channel abnormalities in diabetic cardiomyopathy

One study has described an increase in the number of binding sites for the calcium channel blocker derivative, PH200-110, in the sarcolemmal membrane from diabetic rat hearts [37]. Additionally, data suggest that the action potential may be prolonged in diabetic rat papillary muscles and isolated cardiac myocytes, perhaps as a result of increased calcium currents [38,39]. Action potential prolongation is partly due to decreased outward repolarizing currents, such as the calcium-independent transient outward potassium current (I_{to}) and a reduced quasi–steady-state current [40–42]. This diminished ion channel activity has been correlated with significant reductions in the mRNA of specific potassium channel genes [40]. The action potential duration prolongation seen in diabetic cardiomyopathy results in a suppression of calcium extrusion via sodium-calcium exchange and facilitates the sustained increase in net calcium influx [39]. Depressed sodium-calcium exchange activity has been described in isolated sarcolemmal membranes from diabetic rat hearts [30].

Decreased I_{to} in diabetic myocytes mainly results in a delay in the early phase of repolarization of the cardiac action potential. One consequence of diminished I_{to} in diabetic cardiomyopathy is an increased duration of calcium influx through transmembrane calcium channels [8]. The delayed rectifier current (I_{Kr}) is involved in the slower phase of action potential repolarization. Data suggest that I_{Kr} also is diminished in diabetic cardiomyopathy, and this partially may result in an increased duration of the late repolarization phase of the cardiac action potential [43].

A growing body of evidence suggests that depressed glucose metabolism is a key factor underlying changes in potassium channel function in myocytes from diabetic rat hearts [41,44–46]. Treating isolated ventricular myocytes from diabetic rat hearts with insulin has been shown to upregulate potassium current density back to control levels [41]. Additional evidence suggests that the deleterious effects of diabetes on cardiac potassium channel function involve alterations in cellular redox state [44,47].

Voltage-clamp studies showed that the decreased density of I_{to} in isolated diabetic rat myocytes could be normalized by treatment with insulin (0.1 μM) or the metabolic activator dichloroacetate (1.5 mM) [48]. Inhibitors of glucose-6-phosphate dyhydrogenase, which generates reduced nicotinamide adenine dinucleotide phosphate required by the thioredoxin system, blocked the effect of these agonists on I_{to}. Inhibitors of thioredoxin reductase, which controls the reducing activity of thioredoxin, also blocked the upregulation of I_{to} in response to insulin or dichloroacetate. The results of these studies imply that I_{to} is regulated in a redox-sensitive manner by the thioredoxin system, and that the alterations in I_{to} seen in diabetes may be due to decreased thioredoxin reductase activity [48].

Depressed cardiac sarcoplasmic reticulum function also has been well described in diabetic hearts in several different experimental models. Studies have shown that sarcoplasmic reticulum calcium stores and rates of calcium resequestration into the sarcoplasmic reticulum are significantly reduced in cardiac myocytes from diabetic rats compared with normals [49]. Early data came from isolated cardiac membrane vesicles. In these studies, membranes from diabetic rat hearts showed reduced $^{45}Ca^{2+}$ uptake [27]. More recently, reduced sarcoplasmic reticulum calcium transients have been measured in papillary muscles and isolated cardiac myocytes [32,50]. Caffeine is a known stimulant for sarcoplasmic reticulum calcium release, and the resulting contracture can be used as an indirect measure of the calcium available for release from the sarcoplasmic reticulum. Caffeine-induced calcium transients and contracture are depressed in diabetic myocytes [32,36]. Sarcoplasmic reticulum calcium pump (SERCA) mRNA expression and SERCA activity also were decreased in the left ventricle of rats with dilated cardiomyopathy [51]. Some of these disorders of calcium handling proteins in dilated cardiomyopathy rats reversed with β-blocker treatment [51]; this may explain partially the success of β-blockers in the treatment of cardiomyopathy in diabetic patients.

Renin-angiotensin system in diabetic cardiomyopathy

Activation of the renin-angiotensin system may be a trigger for cardiac myocyte death and contractile dysfunction in diabetic cardiomyopathy. Angiotensin II upregulation also has been implicated in the production of reactive oxygen species, cardiac myocyte loss, and the development of diabetic cardiomyopathy [52]. Upregulation of the renin-angiotensin system may result in diabetic hearts having an increased susceptibility to myocardial ischemia owing to angiotensin II effects on cardiac ion channels. Angiotensin II is a known stimulant of transporters implicated in ischemia-induced calcium overload, including the sodium/hydrogen (Na^+/H^+) exchanger, the sodium/calcium exchanger, and T-type calcium channels [53–55]. Additionally, angiotensin II has been shown to contribute to the activation of protein kinase C-δ, an isoform that has been adversely implicated in the deleterious effects of myocardial ischemia [56].

Hyperglycemic preconditioning is a glucose-mediated protective condition that is associated with increased protein kinase C activity and altered calcium transport that renders myocardial cells resistant to hypoxia. Angiotensin II exposure during prehypoxia blocked this form of cardioprotection in glucose-treated cells [57]. This angiotensin II–mediated blockade of hyperglycemic preconditioning was associated with increased intracellular calcium accumulation during hypoxia, likely mediated via the Na^+/H^+ exchanger and the T-type calcium channel [57]. The Na^+/H^+ exchanger and the T-type calcium channel have been implicated in hypoxia-mediated apoptosis and may account for the deleterious effects of angiotensin II on hypoxic cardiac myocytes.

Treatment of diabetic cardiomyopathy

Several agents have been shown to be beneficial in the treatment of diabetic cardiomyopathy. Treatment with β-blockers, such as carvedilol, has been shown to result in regression of cardiac hypertrophy and an overall decrease in extracellular matrix proteins in diabetic rat hearts [58]. Carvedilol may have additional beneficial effects via its antioxidant, antiproliferative, and hypoglycemic properties [58,59]. Angiotensin-converting enzyme inhibitors, such as captopril, also may be helpful in the treatment of diabetic cardiomyopathy. The angiotensin-converting enzyme inhibitor, captopril, lessens ventricular hypertrophy, decreases capillary network remodeling, and attenuates the proliferation of extracellular matrix proteins seem in diabetic cardiomyopathy [60,61]. Additionally, angiotensin-converting enzyme inhibitors may lessen ischemia-induced calcium overload by blunting angiotensin II–modulated stimulation of processes such as sodium-hydrogen exchange. Short-term treatment with the aldosterone antagonist, spironolactone, may reverse cardiac fibrosis [62].

Insulin-growth factor-I (IGF-I) also may prove useful as a treatment for diabetic cardiomyopathy. IGF-I facilitates glucose metabolism and improves insulin sensitivity [63]. IGF-I has been shown to lessen the contractile abnormalities seen in cardiac myocytes from diabetic rats [2]. Additionally, IGF-I may help restore normal calcium homeostasis in diabetic cardiac myocytes. IGF-I treatment prevents the typical decline in SERCA levels seen in diabetics [64]. IGF-I also has been shown to promote cardiac growth, improve cardiac contractility, and increase cardiac output and ejection volume [2].

Summary

Diabetes mellitus is one of the most common chronic illnesses worldwide. Diabetic cardiomyopathy is a specific syndrome, consisting of cardiomegaly, left ventricular dysfunction, electrical remodeling of the ventricle, and congestive heart failure symptoms, seen in diabetic patients in the absence of other predisposing factors. The etiology of diabetic cardiomyopathy has been linked to a variety of metabolic abnormalities that result in the increased production of reactive oxygen species and depressed myocyte function. A major metabolic abnormality present in patients with diabetic cardiomyopathy is altered calcium homeostasis in cardiac myocytes. This is the result of alterations in the function of various cardiac ion channels, transporters, and exchangers discussed in this article. Treatment with β-blockers, angiotensin-converting enzyme inhibitors, aldosterone antagonists, and perhaps someday novel agents, such as IGF-1, can alter the course of this disease, resulting in improved patient outcome.

References

[1] Janeczko D, Czyzyk A, Kopczynski J, et al. Risk factors of cardiovascular death in diabetic patients. Diabet Med 1991;8(Spec No):S100–3.

[2] Adeghate E. Molecular and cellular basis of the aetiology and management of diabetic cardiomyopathy: a short review. Mol Cell Biochem 2004;261:187–91.

[3] Regan TJ, Lyons MM, Ahmed SS, et al. Evidence for cardiomyopathy in familial diabetes mellitus. J Clin Invest 1977;60:884–99.

[4] Fein FS, Kornstein LB, Strobeck JE, et al. Altered myocardial mechanics in diabetic rats. Circ Res 1980;47:922–33.

[5] Tahiliani AG, McNeill JH. Diabetes-induced abnormalities in the myocardium. Life Sci 1986;38:959–74.

[6] Casis O, Gallego M, Iriarte M, et al. Effects of diabetic cardiomyopathy on regional electrophysiologic characteristics of rat ventricle. Diabetologia 2000;43:101–9.

[7] Shehadeh A, Regan TJ. Cardiac consequences of diabetes mellitus. Clin Cardiol 1995;18: 301–5.

[8] Yu JZ, Rodrigues B, McNeill JH. Intracellular calcium levels are unchanged in the diabetic heart. Cardiovasc Res 1997;34:91–8.

[9] Maritim AC, Sanders RA, Watkins JB 3rd. Diabetes, oxidative stress, and antioxidants: a review. J Biochem Mol Toxicol 2003;17:24–38.

[10] Rodrigues B, Cam MC, McNeill JH. Myocardial substrate metabolism: implications for diabetic cardiomyopathy. J Mol Cell Cardiol 1995;27:169–79.

[11] Cai L, Kang YJ. Oxidative stress and diabetic cardiomyopathy: a brief review. Cardiovasc Toxicol 2001;1:181–93.

[12] Fiordaliso F, Leri A, Cesselli D, et al. Hyperglycemia activates p53 and p53-regulated genes leading to myocyte cell death. Diabetes 2001;50:2363–75.

[13] Kass RS. The channelopathies: novel insights into molecular and genetic mechanisms of human disease. J Clin Invest 2005;115:1986–9.

[14] O'Rourke B, Kass DA, Tomaselli GF, et al. Mechanisms of altered excitation-contraction coupling in canine tachycardia-induced heart failure: I. experimental studies. Circ Res 1999;84:562–70.

[15] Pogwizd SM, Qi M, Yuan W, et al. Upregulation of Na(+)/Ca(2+) exchanger expression and function in an arrhythmogenic rabbit model of heart failure. Circ Res 1999;85:1009–19.

[16] Vadlamudi RV, McNeill JH. Effect of experimental diabetes on rat cardiac cAMP, phosphorylase, and inotropy. Am J Physiol 1983;244:H844–51.

[17] Yu Z, McNeill JH. Altered inotropic responses in diabetic cardiomyopathy and hypertensive-diabetic cardiomyopathy. J Pharmacol Exp Ther 1991;257:64–71.

[18] Dowell RT, Atkins FL, Love S. Integrative nature and time course of cardiovascular alterations in the diabetic rat. J Cardiovasc Pharmacol 1986;8:406–13.

[19] Litwin SE, Raya TE, Anderson PG, et al. Abnormal cardiac function in the streptozotocin-diabetic rat: changes in active and passive properties of the left ventricle. J Clin Invest 1990; 86:481–8.

[20] Kamal AA, Tay SS, Wong WC. The cardiac ganglia in streptozotocin-induced diabetic rats. Arch Histol Cytol 1991;54:41–9.

[21] Lund DD, Subieta AR, Pardini BJ, et al. Alterations in cardiac parasympathetic indices in STZ-induced diabetic rats. Diabetes 1992;41:160–6.

[22] Baandrup U, Ledet T, Rasch R. Experimental diabetic cardiopathy preventable by insulin treatment. Lab Invest 1981;45:169–73.

[23] Sheu SS, Sharma VK, Korth M. Voltage-dependent effects of isoproterenol on cytosolic Ca concentration in rat heart. Am J Physiol 1987;252:H697–703.

[24] Fabiato A. Calcium-induced release of calcium from the cardiac sarcoplasmic reticulum. Am J Physiol 1983;245:C1–14.

[25] Fleischer S, Inui M. Biochemistry and biophysics of excitation-contraction coupling. Annu Rev Biophys Biophys Chem 1989;18:333–64.

[26] Bers DM. Calcium fluxes involved in control of cardiac myocyte contraction. Circ Res 2000; 87:275–81.

[27] Lopaschuk GD, Tahiliani AG, Vadlamudi RV, et al. Cardiac sarcoplasmic reticulum function in insulin- or carnitine-treated diabetic rats. Am J Physiol 1983;245:H969–76.

[28] Dhalla NS, Pierce GN, Innes IR, et al. Pathogenesis of cardiac dysfunction in diabetes mellitus. Can J Cardiol 1985;1:263–81.

[29] Heyliger CE, Prakash A, McNeill JH. Alterations in cardiac sarcolemmal Ca2+ pump activity during diabetes mellitus. Am J Physiol 1987;252:H540–4.

[30] Makino N, Dhalla KS, Elimban V, et al. Sarcolemmal Ca2+ transport in streptozotocin-induced diabetic cardiomyopathy in rats. Am J Physiol 1987;253:E202–7.

[31] Noda N, Hayashi H, Miyata H, et al. Cytosolic Ca2+ concentration and pH of diabetic rat myocytes during metabolic inhibition. J Mol Cell Cardiol 1992;24:435–46.

[32] Yu Z, Tibbits GF, McNeill JH. Cellular functions of diabetic cardiomyocytes: contractility, rapid-cooling contracture, and ryanodine binding. Am J Physiol 1994;266:H2082–9.

[33] Schaffer SW, Mozaffari MS, Artman M, et al. Basis for myocardial mechanical defects associated with non-insulin-dependent diabetes. Am J Physiol 1989;256:E25–30.

[34] Allo SN, Lincoln TM, Wilson GL, et al. Non-insulin-dependent diabetes-induced defects in cardiac cellular calcium regulation. Am J Physiol 1991;260:C1165–71.

[35] Yu Z, Quamme GA, McNeill JH. Depressed [Ca2+]i responses to isoproterenol and cAMP in isolated cardiomyocytes from experimental diabetic rats. Am J Physiol 1994;266: H2334–42.

[36] Yu JZ, Quamme GA, McNeill JH. Altered [Ca2+]i mobilization in diabetic cardiomyocytes: responses to caffeine, KCl, ouabain, and ATP. Diabetes Res Clin Pract 1995;30: 9–20.

[37] Nishio Y, Kashiwagi A, Ogawa T, et al. Increase in [3H]PN 200–110 binding to cardiac muscle membrane in streptozocin-induced diabetic rats. Diabetes 1990;39:1064–9.

[38] Nobe S, Aomine M, Arita M, et al. Chronic diabetes mellitus prolongs action potential duration of rat ventricular muscles: circumstantial evidence for impaired Ca2+ channel. Cardiovasc Res 1990;24:381–9.

[39] Shigematsu S, Maruyama T, Kiyosue T, et al. Rate-dependent prolongation of action potential duration in single ventricular myocytes obtained from hearts of rats with streptozotocin-induced chronic diabetes sustained for 30–32 weeks. Heart Vessels 1994;9:300–6.

[40] Qin D, Huang B, Deng L, et al. Downregulation of K(+) channel genes expression in type I diabetic cardiomyopathy. Biochem Biophys Res Commun 2001;283:549–53.

[41] Shimoni Y, Ewart HS, Severson D. Insulin stimulation of rat ventricular K+ currents depends on the integrity of the cytoskeleton. J Physiol 1999;514(Pt 3):735–45.

[42] Shimoni Y, Chuang M, Abel ED, et al. Gender-dependent attenuation of cardiac potassium currents in type 2 diabetic db/db mice. J Physiol 2004;555:345–54.

[43] Jourdon P, Feuvray D. Calcium and potassium currents in ventricular myocytes isolated from diabetic rats. J Physiol 1993;470:411–29.

[44] Rozanski GJ, Xu Z. A metabolic mechanism for cardiac K+ channel remodelling. Clin Exp Pharmacol Physiol 2002;29:132–7.

[45] Xu Z, Patel KP, Rozanski GJ. Intracellular protons inhibit transient outward K+ current in ventricular myocytes from diabetic rats. Am J Physiol 1996;271:H2154–61.

[46] Xu Z, Patel KP, Rozanski GJ. Metabolic basis of decreased transient outward K+ current in ventricular myocytes from diabetic rats. Am J Physiol 1996;271:H2190–6.

[47] Xu Z, Patel KP, Lou MF, et al. Up-regulation of K(+) channels in diabetic rat ventricular myocytes by insulin and glutathione. Cardiovasc Res 2002;53:80–8.

[48] Li X, Xu Z, Li S, et al. Redox regulation of Ito remodeling in diabetic rat heart. Am J Physiol Heart Circ Physiol 2005;288:H1417–24.

[49] Choi KM, Zhong Y, Hoit BD, et al. Defective intracellular Ca(2+) signaling contributes to cardiomyopathy in Type 1 diabetic rats. Am J Physiol Heart Circ Physiol 2002;283: H1398–408.

[50] Bouchard RA, Bose D. Influence of experimental diabetes on sarcoplasmic reticulum function in rat ventricular muscle. Am J Physiol 1991;260:H341–54.

[51] Zhang JN, Geng Q, Chen XJ, et al. Alteration of endothelin system and calcium handling protein in left ventricles following drug treatment in dilated cardiomyopathy rats. Acta Pharmacol Sin 2003;24:1099–102.

[52] Fiordaliso F, Li B, Latini R, et al. Myocyte death in streptozotocin-induced diabetes in rats in angiotensin II-dependent. Lab Invest 2000;80:513–27.

[53] Ballard C, Schaffer S. Stimulation of the Na+/Ca2+ exchanger by phenylephrine, angiotensin II and endothelin 1. J Mol Cell Cardiol 1996;28:11–7.

[54] Ferron L, Capuano V, Ruchon Y, et al. Angiotensin II signaling pathways mediate expression of cardiac T-type calcium channels. Circ Res 2003;93:1241–8.

[55] Gunasegaram S, Haworth RS, Hearse DJ, et al. Regulation of sarcolemmal Na(+)/H(+) exchanger activity by angiotensin II in adult rat ventricular myocytes: opposing actions via AT(1) versus AT(2) receptors. Circ Res 1999;85:919–30.

[56] Murriel CL, Mochly-Rosen D. Opposing roles of delta and epsilonPKC in cardiac ischemia and reperfusion: targeting the apoptotic machinery. Arch Biochem Biophys 2003;420: 246–54.

[57] Pastukh V, Wu S, Ricci C, et al. Reversal of hyperglycemic preconditioning by angiotensin II: role of calcium transport. Am J Physiol Heart Circ Physiol 2005;288:H1965–75.

[58] Grimm D, Jabusch HC, Kossmehl P, et al. Experimental diabetes and left ventricular hypertrophy: effects of beta-receptor blockade. Cardiovasc Pathol 2002;11:229–37.

[59] Bril A, Slivjak M, DiMartino MJ, et al. Cardioprotective effects of carvedilol, a novel beta adrenoceptor antagonist with vasodilating properties, in anaesthetised minipigs: comparison with propranolol. Cardiovasc Res 1992;26:518–25.

[60] Al-Shafei AI, Wise RG, Gresham GA, et al. Non-invasive magnetic resonance imaging assessment of myocardial changes and the effects of angiotensin-converting enzyme inhibition in diabetic rats. J Physiol 2002;538:541–53.

[61] Sugawara T, Fujii S, Akm Zaman T, et al. Coronary capillary remodeling in non-insulin-dependent diabetic rats: amelioration by inhibition of angiotensin converting enzyme and its potential clinical implications. Hypertens Res 2001;24:75–81.

[62] Miric G, Dallemagne C, Endre Z, et al. Reversal of cardiac and renal fibrosis by pirfenidone and spironolactone in streptozotocin-diabetic rats. Br J Pharmacol 2001;133:687–94.

[63] Ren J, Samson WK, Sowers JR. Insulin-like growth factor I as a cardiac hormone: physio-logical and pathophysiological implications in heart disease. J Mol Cell Cardiol 1999;31: 2049–61.
[64] Norby FL, Wold LE, Duan J, et al. IGF-I attenuates diabetes-induced cardiac contractile dysfunction in ventricular myocytes. Am J Physiol Endocrinol Metab 2002;283:E658–66.

ELSEVIER
SAUNDERS

Endocrinol Metab Clin N Am
35 (2006) 611–631

ENDOCRINOLOGY
AND METABOLISM
CLINICS
OF NORTH AMERICA

Polycystic Ovarian Syndrome: the Next Cardiovascular Dilemma in Women?

Preethi Srikanthan, MD[a], Stanley Korenman, MD[b],
Susan Davis, MD[b],*

[a]Department of Epidemiology and Preventative Medicine,
University of California Los Angeles, Box 957065, 330 South Garfield Avenue,
Suite 308, Los Angeles, CA 90095, USA
[b]Department of Endocrinology, Diabetes and Metabolism,
University of California Los Angeles, Box 951680, 52-242 CHS, Los Angeles, CA 90095, USA

The polycystic ovary syndrome (PCOS), which features amenorrhea, hirsutism, and obesity, affects 10% of the female population [1,2], representing 7 to 10 million women (of reproductive age) in the United States. It was described histologically by Stein and Leventhal [3] in 1935 and initially treated as a reproductive and cosmetic concern of young reproductive-age women, but more recently PCOS has been recognized to have metabolic and cardiovascular associations that make it of major consequence for women of all ages worldwide. The increased prevalence of insulin resistance, impaired glucose tolerance, type 2 diabetes, dyslipidemia, and several cardiovascular risk factors has elevated PCOS from a surgical curiosity to a metabolic derangement with significant public health ramifications. The heterogeneity of the phenotypes (clinically and biochemically) leads to difficulty in achieving a precise diagnosis, defining a single underlying pathogenesis, and selecting a homogeneous population for much needed prospective studies. Insulin resistance is an aspect of the pathophysiology of PCOS that predisposes these women to developing several cardiovascular risk factors.

Dilemmas in definition

PCOS has lacked a precise and uniform definition. One more recent attempt at establishing diagnostic criteria, formulated in a 1990 National Institute of Child Health and Human Development consensus conference on

---

* Corresponding author. Santa Monica Community Practice, 1801 Wilshire Boulevard, Suite 100, Santa Monica, CA 90403, USA.
E-mail address: ssdavis@mednet.ucla.edu (S. Davis).

0889-8529/06/$ - see front matter © 2006 Elsevier Inc. All rights reserved.
doi:10.1016/j.ecl.2006.05.001

polycystic ovary syndrome (PCOS), included chronic anovulation and bio-chemically or clinically evident hyperandrogenism. The 2003 Rotterdam consensus workshop on PCOS [4] added an ultrasound description, supple-menting, rather than more precisely defining, the condition (Box 1).

Both definitions in Box 1 leave room for clinical, biochemical, and hor-monal heterogeneity. Levels of biochemically significant hyperandrogenism are not defined and globally accepted [5], and similarly there is no agreement on normal versus abnormal age-appropriate levels of androstenedione and dihydroepiandrosterone sulfate (DHEAS). Oligo-ovulation and anovulation also need better clinical or biochemical definition (or both) [6]. Irregular uterine bleeding is common, and fewer than eight menses per year is com-monly accepted as oligomenorrhea, but this can vary. Some patients may have regular menses intermittently; some patients, with hirsutism and re-ported "regular" menses, may be anovulatory with low luteal phase proges-terone. The radiologic criteria for ultrasound definition of PCOS are not commonly used (increased ovarian volume $> 10 \text{ cm}^3$ or at least 12 follicular cysts measuring 2–9 mm or both [7]). More recent studies have attempted to discern subcategories of PCOS patients. Carmina and coworkers [6] divided a group of women who presented for evaluation of clinical hyperandrogen-ism and were biochemically hyperandrogenic into the following three categories:

1. Hyperandrogenism with chronic anovulation (classic PCOS)
2. Hyperandrogenism with normal ovulatory cycles, but polycystic ovaries on ultrasound (ovulatory PCOS)
3. Idiopathic hyperandrogenic patients with normal cycles and normal ul-trasound appearance of ovaries (idiopathic hyperandrogenic).

Box 1. Criteria for polycystic ovary syndrome

1990 National Institutes of Health criteria for PCOS
2 out of 2 of the following:
   1. Chronic anovulation
   2. Clinical or biochemical signs of hyperandrogenism
Exclusion of other causes

2003 Rotterdam criteria for PCOS
2 out of 3 of the following:
   1. Oligo-ovulation or anovulation
   2. Clinical or biochemical signs of hyperandrogenism
   3. Polycystic ovaries
Exclusion of other causes (congenital adrenal hyperplasia, androgen-secreting tumors, Cushing's syndrome, thyroid disease, prolactinoma)

Carmina and coworkers [6] were able to establish a difference in metabolic characteristics in these subcategories, including a hierarchy of prevalence of risk factors (including insulin resistance, dyslipidemia, homocysteine, and C-reactive protein [CRP]) such that:

Classic PCOS > ovulatory PCOS > idiopathic hyperandrogenic

Establishing subcategories may lead to a clearer definition of a woman's level of metabolic and cardiovascular risk. More important, clinicians must look at each woman's risk profile of developing cardiovascular disease, whatever her PCOS phenotype.

Pathophysiologies of polycystic ovary syndrome

Hyperandrogenism is important in the development of PCOS, but insulin resistance (and hyperinsulinism) is detectable early in the development of PCOS and may be crucial to the development of those aspects of PCOS that predispose to cardiovascular disease.

Hyperandrogenemia

One of the most recognizable and expressed traits is hyperandrogenism; two thirds of classic PCOS patients have hirsutism or its equivalents, including acne, oily skin, and alopecia. The hyperandrogenemia seems to be of ovarian and adrenal origin. This disordered steroid biosynthesis was identified by Ehrmann and colleagues [8], who showed elevated ovarian and adrenal C-19 precursors (Fig. 1).

The functional ovarian hyperandrogenism is gonadotropin dependent, suppressible by long-term estrogen/progestin or gonadotropin therapy, but not glucocorticoid therapy [8–10]. Evidence for a primary ovarian cause of hyperandogenism is seen in the persistence of abnormal steroidogenesis through multiple cell passages of cultured ovarian thecal cells [11]. Oral contraceptive pills reliably lower bioavailable testosterone levels to low-normal and improve the cosmetic and irregularity problems; the clinical importance of ovarian hyperandrogenism and its therapy should be emphasized.

Increased frequency of hypothalamic release of gonadotropin-releasing hormone (GnRH) is found in women with PCOS. GnRH pulses determine the ratio of luteinizing hormone (LH) to follicle-stimulating hormone (FSH) synthesis by pituitary gonadotropes so that LH pulses also are increased in frequency and amplitude. Elevated LH levels and LH-to-FSH ratio greater than 3 are seen in 66% of patients. The PCOS ovary responds to the increased LH stimulation with increased ovarian androgen production. Progestin normally slows the GnRH pulse release, but there is a decline in progestin with decreased ovulatory events in PCOS. Low progesterone, with tonic hyperestrogenism, enhances gonadotroph sensitivity to GnRH,

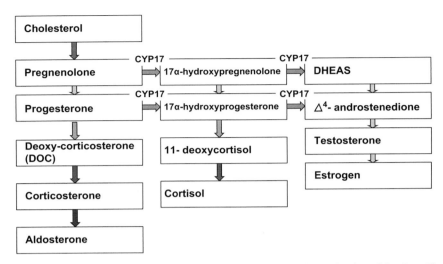

Fig. 1. Pathway of steroid biosynthesis. Abnormalities favoring the production of the three 19-carbon principal androgens (dihydroepiandrosterone [DHEA], DHEAS, and Δ-4-androstene-dione) occur in PCOS. Androgens are steroids with 19 carbon atoms, located in the biosynthesis chain between progestins and estrogens. The main androgen is testosterone, which is formed by the peripheral interconversion product of Δ-4-androstenedione, whose origin is mixed, from the ovary and the cortex of the adrenals. DHEA essentially comes from the adrenals and is accumulated in the form of a sulfate, DHEAS. In PCOS, there is thought to be increased activity of CYP17, leading to increased C 19 steroids accumulation. (CYP17 = P450c17.)

resulting in increased LH release. A vicious cycle involving oligo-ovulation leading to increased frequency of GnRH pulses leading to increased LH, decreased cycles, and increased androgens may be perpetuated prepubertally.

Insulin and insulin-like growth factor-1 also have been shown to stimulate theca interstitial cells to produce androgen. They prime theca cells for LH-stimulated androgen synthesis and suppress steroid hormone–binding globulin (SHBG) production from human hepatoma cell lines [12]. Insulin and insulin-like growth factor-1 have been shown to be elevated in PCOS subjects and in patients with polycystic-appearing ovaries on ultrasound [13], and the insulin-like growth factor binding protein-1 levels are correspondingly decreased.

Hyperinsulinemia has been blamed for triggering production of excess androgens [14,15], but this is an inconsistent finding [16]. Nestler and coworkers [15] noted that after administration of oral diazoxide, there was not only a significant decrease in serum insulin, but also a concomitant significant decrease in serum total testosterone with a nonsignificant increase in serum SHBG. Conversion of the excess androgen (androstenedione) to estrone occurs peripherally. Estrone levels are normal to increased in women with PCOS. Estradiol levels are usually normal, but as a result of the reduced SHBG, free estradiol may be high. These sustained levels of estrogen may cause endometrial hyperplasia and the increased risk of endometrial carcinoma found in women with PCOS. A few patients also have mild hyperprolactinemia (<40 ng/mL) as a result of estrogenic lactotroph stimulation. Hyperandrogenism clusters in families and seems to be genetic, with studies showing that even male family members of PCOS patients exhibit elevated DHEAS levels [17,18].

Hyperinsulinemia and insulin resistance

Hyperinsulinemia initially was described in women with PCOS by several groups [19], all of whom noted that in nonobese PCOS patients there was more insulin resistance compared with normal ovulating controls. Despite the use of many different techniques to measure insulin resistance, it is identified in no more than 60% of PCOS subjects.

Insulin resistance does seem to be important in the orchestration of many events in the development of PCOS, including the following:

- Stimulation of ovarian androgen production [14,15,20]
- Induction of ovarian LH receptors [21]
- Decreasing insulin-like growth factor binding protein-1 production and increasing free insulin-like growth factor-1, which stimulates proliferation of thecal cells [22]
- Stimulation of pituitary LH secretion, upregulating testosterone production [23]

The cause of insulin resistance in PCOS is likely multifactorial related to one or more of several factors discussed next.

Obesity

Obesity is present in at least 30% PCOS patients, and in some series, the percentage is 75% [24], with women with PCOS in the United States having a generally higher body weight than their European counterparts [6]. In the United States, there has been a gradual increase in incidence of PCOS that parallels the increase in obesity [25] and type 2 diabetes.

The distribution of adiposity may have differential effects on development of features of PCOS. The presence of fat accumulation in the upper body (android fat pattern) is associated with an increased incidence of hyperandrogenism [26] and diminishing fertility [27], and this body phenotype has been noted in obese and lean women with PCOS [28–30]. Distribution of body fat in the lower body regions (gynoid fat pattern) evolves during normal female puberty and is associated with a regular ovulatory menstrual cycle and fertility [31]. Additionally, it has been noted that women with an android fat pattern are at inherent risk for developing cardiovascular disease and diabetes mellitus type 2 [32]. Weight loss has been noted to result in significant reduction in androgen concentrations and blood glucose and insulin concentrations in obese women who do not have PCOS [33] and even more consistently in obese PCOS patients [34]. Insulin sensitivity does not have a linear relationship with body mass index (BMI) per se, and it is influenced by the distribution of adipose tissue to a greater degree than genetics, age, exercise (chronic or acute), or diet [35].

Obese women with PCOS have higher mean fasting insulin levels and greater insulin response to glucose challenge. These obese PCOS patients had lower insulin sensitivity by several different assessment techniques, including quantitative insulin sensitivity check index, fasting glucose to insulin ratio, and insulin sensitivity index [13]. Goodarzi and coworkers [36] compared results from 69 PCOS patients with National Health and Nutrition Examination Survey (NHANES) II data. Analysis of insulin sensitivity, blood pressure, lipid profiles, and androgen levels in these PCOS patients determined that the most insulin-resistant tertile of patients exhibited higher BMI, androgen levels, systolic and diastolic blood pressure, triglyceride levels, and decreased high-density lipoprotein (HDL) cholesterol levels, relating insulin resistance to obesity.

Similarly, in a study of 24 obese patients (mean weight 91.5 kg [SD 14.7 kg]) placed on a 1000-Kcal diet for 6 to 7 months [37], it was noted that 13 women lost greater than 5% of their original body weight. Forty percent of these women had a reduction in hirsutism and reduction in fasting serum insulin levels. Nine women had an improvement in reproductive function (ie, five conceived, and the others regularized their periods). Because not all women with PCOS are obese, however, the greater degree of insulin resistance described in PCOS patients may be caused by other factors and exacerbated by obesity in some.

Androgens

Whether hyperandrogenism contributes to the insulin resistance is less clear. Diamond and colleagues [38] studied regularly menstruating, nonobese women before and during methyltestosterone administration (5 mg three times a day for 10–12 days) and showed that short-term androgen excess led to decreased insulin-stimulated glucose uptake. Carmina and coworkers [6] claimed that all their hyperandrogenic subjects showed some degree of insulin resistance, whereas the hyperandrogenic subjects with polycystic ovaries were most insulin resistant.

Dunaif and associates [39] were unable to confirm a cause-and-effect relationship between hyperandrogenism and insulin resistance when they administered a GnRH analogue to PCOS patients. Despite significant decreases in plasma testosterone and androstenedione levels caused by the analogue, there was no significant change in insulin-mediated glucose disposal, plasma insulin levels, or hepatic glucose production.

Intrinsic carbohydrate regulation system abnormalities

In PCOS, insulin binding seems to be normal, but there is a defect in post receptor signal transduction [40]. The above-noted factors act at one of the levels of the insulin signaling pathway, resulting in insulin resistance. Some possible post insulin receptor signaling abnormalities are discussed next.

Rosenbaum and coworkers [41] noted insulin-stimulated glucose transport declined by 40% in obese patients and 36% in PCOS patients (independent of obesity) compared with lean normal patients. A decline in cell surface glucose transporter-4 (GLUT-4) content was found in obese and PCOS patients.

In vitro studies have shown that serine phosphorylation of the β subunit of the insulin receptor causes insulin receptor inactivation and insulin resistance [42]. Serine phosphorylation also may lead to hyperandrogenemia via hyperphosphorylation of the steroidogenic enzyme P450c17, which catalyzes scission of the C17-C20 steroid bond (17,20-lyase) and increases C-19 steroid synthesis (see Fig. 1) [43]. A gain-of-function mutation in cyclic adenosine monophosphate–inducible serine kinase potentially could relate the insulin resistance and hyperandrogenism in some families [43].

Genetics

Although no one specific insulin signaling mutation has been identified, genetic studies do show familial incidence of PCOS [44]. Insulin resistance is found in sisters of women with PCOS and increased insulin levels, insulin resistance and glucose tolerance were found in first-degree relatives of another series of PCOS patients. Brothers of PCOS patients were noted to have insulin resistance and endothelial dysfunction [46], in addition to the increased DHEAS levels reported in male relatives [11].

Risk factors for cardiovascular disease in polycystic ovary syndrome

Increased cardiovascular risk may be expected in women with PCOS because of its association with the prevalence of several risk factors [14], including insulin resistance, impaired glucose tolerance (IGT), type 2 diabetes, hypertension, dyslipidemia, coagulopathy (elevated plasminogen activator inhibitor 1[PAI-1], decreased fibrinolytic activity, and platelet dysfunction), chronic inflammation (CRP), homocysteine and abnormal adipokines, endothelial dysfunction, sleep apnea, and genetic/ethnic predisposition (Table 1). Sam and Dunaif [47] believed the most significant determinant of cardiovascular disease in PCOS patients is insulin resistance, and PCOS may be viewed as another metabolic syndrome equivalent, leading them to call PCOS syndrome XX. The prevalence of the metabolic syndrome is increased twofold in PCOS patients compared with age-matched women [48]. Based on a risk factor model for myocardial infarction in PCOS patients, using the prevalence of some of the known risk factors, predictions of a sevenfold increase in relative risk for myocardial infarction have been made [49].

Childhood antecedents of PCOS have been found, and by adolescence these patients develop many of the cardiovascular risk factor patterns

Table 1
Distribution of risk factors in cardiovascular disease and polycystic ovary syndrome

Risk factor	Effect in PCOS	Reference
Insulin resistance	Increased	[47]
Hypertension	Increased	[51]
Endothelial dysfunction	Increased	[62]
Dyslipidemia	Increased triglyceride, LDL	[56]
	Decreased HDL	
Endothelin 1	Increased	[61]
PAI-1	Increased	[72]
Homocysteine	Increased	[84]
CRP	Increased	[88]
Adipokines	Increased resistin	[107]
	Decreased adiponectin	
Obesity	Increased	[24]

shared by women with PCOS [50]. Dahlgren and coworkers [51], in a study of 33 PCOS patients who had undergone wedge resection for PCOS 22 to 30 years before, noted that women with PCOS continue to have a significantly greater incidence of hypertension, diabetes, basal insulin, and waist-to-hip ratio.

Insulin resistance, impaired glucose tolerance and diabetes mellitus type 2

Insulin resistance, IGT, and diabetes mellitus type 2 are among the most important risk factors for cardiovascular disease found with increased frequency in women with PCOS. Insulin-resistant individuals are at greater risk of developing not only PCOS, but also IGT and diabetes type 2, essential hypertension, nonalcoholic steatohepatitis, dyslipidemia, sleep apnea, and certain cancers [52]. Although insulin resistance is not proven to be an independent predictor of cardiovascular disease, it is associated (as shown by the previous list) with known cardiovascular risk factors.

In one US study, approximately 40% to 45% of PCOS patients had IGT or frank type 2 diabetes, whereas 69% of PCOS patients had insulin resistance [44]. Ehrmann and colleagues [53], using an oral glucose tolerance test in 122 women with PCOS, showed the prevalence of IGT was 35% and type 2 diabetes was 10%, higher than in age-matched and weight-matched women without PCOS. It seems that many PCOS patients with insulin resistance alone are able to compensate sufficiently, whereas other PCOS patients (especially patients with a first-degree relative with type 2 diabetes) also have an impaired β cell response to meals and glucose challenge [54] and develop IGT and diabetes mellitus type 2. Given that prediabetes and diabetes are well-established cardiovascular disease risks [55], determination of insulin sensitivity and glucose tolerance should be an essential component of the workup of PCOS patients.

Hypertension and endothelial dysfunction

It has been found that the 50% of hypertensive patients who also have insulin resistance have the greatest risk of cardiovascular disease [56]. Arslanian and coworkers [57] noted an absence of the nocturnal dip in blood pressure in young teenagers with PCOS, suggesting the early onset of blood pressure dysregulation. The Nurses' Health Study data showed that a longer, or irregular, menstrual cycle length led to a twofold increase in risk of hypertension in such women [58]. Although Dahlgren and associates [51] reported an incidence of hypertension of 39% in PCOS patients compared with 11% in age-matched controls, Talbott and coworkers [59] found no such differences after adjusting for BMI.

Hypertension in women with PCOS reflects abnormalities in vascular compliance and vascular endothelial function that have been noted in several studies [60–62]. Kravariti and colleagues [63] studied endothelial function in 62 women with PCOS who were divided into three groups of lean, overweight, and obese. Impaired vascular compliance was more than could be predicted by obesity alone [60], but seemed to be related to insulin resistance. They found insulin resistance, total testosterone, and total cholesterol were independent predictors of endothelial dysfunction, accounting for 21%, 10%, and 9% of the variance ($P < .005$ for all). Insulin sensitizers, including troglitazone [64] and metformin [65], led to an improvement of endothelial dysfunction. Other groups have reported similar findings of significantly impaired endothelial function in young nonobese PCOS patients [61,66]. Endothelin-1 is increased in PCOS patients [67]. In vitro, endothelin-1 gene expression is increased by exposing endothelial cells to high concentrations of insulin [68], linking PCOS and hyperinsulinemia to endothelial dysfunction.

Coagulopathy

Disorders of coagulation occur in and contribute to atherosclerosis [69,70], and several groups now are evaluating the pathophysiology of coagulation dysfunction in PCOS patients. Dereli and coworkers [71] evaluated agonist-induced platelet aggregation in 50 women with PCOS, 50 women with nonclassic congenital adrenal hyperplasia, and 30 women in a control group. Platelet hyperaggregation was seen only in the women with PCOS, not noted in hyperandrogenic patients with nonclassic congenital adrenal hyperplasia, which suggests that the hyperaggregation in PCOS may be due to the insulin resistance. Macut and coworkers [72] noted that obese

PCOS patients had higher PAI-1 levels than in control subjects. PAI-1 levels were even higher in women with PCOS than in type 2 diabetes patients [73], and the PAI-1 concentration maybe reduced with metformin therapy [74].

Dyslipidemia

Hypertension and dyslipidemia are found to be significantly increased in PCOS patients and their first-degree relatives [75]. An atherogenic lipid profile contributes to concerns of vascular disease in PCOS patients. In addition to increased very low-density lipoprotein (VLDL), increased low-density lipoprotein (LDL), and decreased high-density lipoprotein (HDL), hypertriglyceridemia is found with hyperandrogenism and insulin resistance [59]. Low HDL levels in PCOS patients, have been most associated commonly with obesity, whereas high LDL levels are better related to hyperandrogenemia [76,77]. These results persist even after adjusting for BMI [59]. Hyperandrogenism and insulin resistance contribute to this pattern of dyslipidemia in PCOS. Finally, lipoprotein lipase activity is decreased in abdominal adipocytes by dihydrotestosterone [78].

Adipokines

Along with recognition of the adipocyte as an endocrine organ has come understanding that abnormal production of adipokines may contribute to cardiovascular risk [79]. Elevated resistin and low adiponectin levels have been found in patients with PCOS and their mothers and fathers, possibly contributing to increased cardiovascular disease risk [45]. In a study of 55 patients with PCOS and 45 normally ovulating controls, adiponectin was lower and resistin higher in the PCOS patients, with this relationship persisting in the case of adiponectin levels after controlling for BMI [80]. Visceral adiposity may be of particular concern, but has not been well studied.

Markers of inflammation

Homocysteine

Hyperhomocysteinemia is associated with adverse cardiovascular outcomes [81,82]. Lowering the plasma homocysteine improves endothelial function in patients with coronary artery disease, resulting in decreased incidence of cardiovascular events [83]. In the PCOS population, several groups have noted increased homocysteine levels in PCOS patients. Yilmaz and coworkers [84] noted that hyperhomocysteinemia is present to a greater degree in obese and nonobese PCOS patients than in healthy weight-matched controls. The increase in homocysteine was independent of serum insulin levels and the BMI. Interventions known to improve insulin sensitivity and decrease progression from obesity to type 2 diabetes, including exercise/ lifestyle change [85] and metformin use [86], have been noted, however, to decrease homocysteine in PCOS patients. Hyperhomocysteinemia may be an independent risk, additive to insulin resistance and obesity, in PCOS patients predisposing to cardiovascular disease.

C-reactive protein

CRP has been associated with cardiovascular disease [87], and its increase in patients with PCOS may reflect increased risk in these women. CRP levels were significantly higher in obese PCOS patients at baseline and significantly decreased with metformin therapy in a study of 52 PCOS patients (32 obese and 20 nonobese) randomized to receive metformin or Diane (ethinyl estradiol/cyproterone) for 3 months [88].

Genetics

Ethnic variation exists in the clinical features and biochemical abnormalities of PCOS. Rodin and colleagues [89] noted in a community study in Britain that the highest prevalence of PCOS was in South Asian immigrants (52%). In this group of PCOS patients, there was a degree of insulin resistance comparable to age-matched South Asian women with established type 2 diabetes without PCOS. Cardiovascular disease burden is high in this community [90]. Finally, patients with PCOS have more family history of coronary artery disease, as noted by Kaushal [46] in the brothers of PCOS patients.

Evidence for increased cardiovascular risk in polycystic ovary syndrome—is the jury still out?

There is currently no definitive answer to the question whether PCOS independently leads to cardiovascular disease. One reason is that these women often are studied when young, long before cardiovascular disease occurs. To deal with this problem, Pierpoint and coworkers [91] studied 786 women with PCOS who underwent wedge resection between 1930 and 1979. These patients seemed to have no increase in cardiovascular mortality compared with expected, age-specific and sex-specific mortality rates in the United Kingdom. In a follow-up study [92], in which the cohort was sent questionnaires, it was found that the odds ratio for coronary heart disease was 1.5 (although this was not statistically significant because it was based only on 15 cardiovascular events in the PCOS group), with a similarly increased (although statistically significant) odds ratio of 2.8 for cerebrovascular disease. In the British study (and in several other observational studies of PCOS patients), the control group had a higher BMI. Ensuring a comparable BMI is important, and perhaps the distribution of adipose tissue (the significance of which was discussed earlier in the section on obesity) should be considered in PCOS and control groups.

Using the Nurses' Health Study database, Solomon and coworkers [93] reported an adjusted relative risk of 1.53 (95% confidence interval 1.24–1.90) for coronary heart disease in women with a history of irregular menstrual cycles, which was used as a marker of PCOS. In a nested case control in the Women's Health Study database, lower SHBG and higher calculated free androgen index (suggesting that they were PCOS patients) were noted in the women who developed cardiovascular events [94]. Cibula and associates [95] found a fourfold higher risk of cardiovascular disease over a 20-year follow-up period. A prospective study analyzing cardiovascular outcomes and effects of treatment of PCOS patients is awaited.

Evidence for vascular disease in PCOS patients, as a precursor of atherosclerosis, has been shown using various imaging modalities. Guzick [96] noted that the carotid intimal medial thickness (IMT) was significantly greater in 16 PCOS patients compared with 16 controls. The IMT result was associated significantly with insulin, total cholesterol, LDL levels, and BMI of the patients, as could be expected from aforementioned studies. It has been suggested, however, that the relationship between PCOS and vascular disease may not be so simple. Talbott and coworkers [97], in a study of 47 PCOS patients who underwent carotid ultrasound, noted that obesity partially explained the influence of PCOS on IMT. The effect of BMI on the PCOS-IMT relationship was not completely determined by hyperinsulinemia or visceral fat and might be mediated by other aspects of PCOS-related adiposity.

Coronary artery calcification (CAC) assessed by noninvasive electron beam tomography correlates with the degree of atherosclerosis found on pathologic examination and predicts incident cardiovascular events. Talbott and coworkers [98] noted that women with PCOS had a higher prevalence of coronary artery calcium (45.9% versus 30.6%) than controls. After adjustment for age and BMI, PCOS was a significant predictor of CAC (odds ratio 2.31; $P = .049$). A similar result was obtained in a study by Christian and colleagues [99], who noted CAC was more prevelant in women with PCOS (39%) than in age-matched and weight-matched controls (21%; $P = .05$) or community-dwelling women (9.9%; $P < .001$), suggesting increased risk of atheroscerosis in PCOS patients.

Orio and coworkers [100] noted in a study of 30 PCOS women and 30 age-matched and BMI-matched controls that compared with echocardiographic evaluations of asymptomatic lean women with PCOS, there was increased left atrial size, left ventricular mass index and left ventricular ejection fraction (among other parameters). Diastolic dysfunction has been noted with increased prevalence in women with PCOS [101,102].

Wild and associates [103] found more atherosclerosis on coronary catheterization of hirsute women compared with controls. In a study of 143 women (age ≤ 60 years) who had had coronary angiography, women with more extensive coronary artery disease (number of segments with $> 50\%$ stenosis) were more likely than women with less extensive disease to have polycystic ovaries on ultrasound and other distinct metabolic and endocrine abnormalities, such as higher free testosterone, higher triglycerides, lower HDL, and higher C-peptide levels [104].

Finally, as noted by Legro [105] in a review of this topic, there are several major impediments to completing adequate trials to assess whether PCOS patients are at increased risk for cardiovascular disease. There is such diversity of phenotypes of PCOS and modality and duration of therapies that it is difficult to gather a homogeneous group of PCOS participants for assessment of cardiovascular disease risk. If medication is chosen to correct risk factors or improve insulin sensitivity, it may be needed for life. Clear outcomes studies are important. Despite the proliferation of PCOS studies using risk factors or surrogate cardiovascular end points, hard end points are required to prove causality, as clinicians well know from the example of hormone replacement therapy and its lack of a role in cardiovascular protection.

Who, what, and how to screen

The American College of Cardiologists advises screening women in general for the presence of the following established risk factors: smoking, diabetes, hypertension, obesity, elevated serum LDL cholesterol, and low serum HDL cholesterol. In women with PCOS, clinicians also should look more closely for metabolic derangements with fasting glucose and insulin levels, hemoglobin A_{1c}, lipid subfractions, a 2-hour oral glucose tolerance test, or 2-hour postprandial glucose level, in addition to diagnostic medical laboratory tests including bioavailable testosterone, DHEAS, 17-hydroxycorticosteroid progesterone, thyrotropin, and prolactin. When clinically indicated, a 24-hour urine free cortisol or cosyntropin (Cortrosyn) stimulation test also might be done.

PCOS patients with central obesity, features of metabolic syndrome, and insulin resistance seem to be most likely to develop the complications of glucose intolerance/type 2 diabetes and cardiovascular disease. Clinicians should screen and treat these patients most intensely. All of these patients should be monitored periodically with postprandial glucose and fasting lipids in addition to addressing their concerns with hirsutism, menstruation, or fertility.

Formal assessment of insulin resistance is supported only in the context of a clinical study. The clinical response to insulin-lowering therapies does not seem to be related to the magnitude of insulin resistance, and there may be little gained by formal measurement of insulin sensitivity in PCOS patients. The finding of increased cardiovascular disease in first-degree family members by Yilmaz [45] suggests that clinicians should be screening PCOS patients and their families for metabolic abnormalities and cardiovascular risk factors.

Therapies that address cardiovascular risk

Table 2 summarizes therapies for PCOS.

Weight loss and exercise

Lifestyle modification, which accomplished a 7% weight loss by diet and 150 minutes of physical activity per week, improved insulin sensitivity and decreased progression to type 2 diabetes in the Diabetes Prevention Program [106]. Weight loss in type 2 diabetic patients lowered hemoglobin A_{1c}, blood pressure, total cholesterol and triglycerides, and elevated HDL levels. Diet and weight loss improved hirsutism and menstrual disorders in women with PCOS, and not only did androgen levels decline, but also glucose and insulin concentrations decreased [34]. Many women who lost greater than 5% of original body weight showed improved ovulation, and some conceived [37]. Any method of weight loss may accomplish similar benefits. Orlistat and acarbose-induced weight loss in obese PCOS patients have been shown to lower free androgens, increase SHBG, and improve hirsutism and menstrual patterns [107].

Metformin

Metformin improves insulin sensitivity and hyperandrogenemia in PCOS patients. Additionally, several studies have shown that metformin use leads to changes in other factors in PCOS patients, such as systolic blood pressure (decreased), apolipoprotien A-I (increased) [74], adiponectin (increased), and endothelial dysfunction (improved). In one study [108], metformin and rosiglitazone therapy (in women with PCOS) was noted to cause a significant increase in mean plasma homocysteine, while increasing apolipoprotein A-I, and decreasing total cholesterol, HDL, and LDL. When folic acid and vitamin B were administered with metformin, the negative outcomes were averted. This study typifies the general need for large prospective studies

Table 2
Treatments for polycystic ovary syndrome

Treatment	Mode of action	Indications
Weight loss/diet control	Improve insulin sensitivity Influence regular ovulatory cycle commencement	BMI >25, IGT
Oral contraceptive pills	Reduce LH-stimulated androgens Increase SHBG, reduce free androgens	Reproductive-age women needing contraception
Antiandrogens	Androgen receptor blockade 5α-reductase inhibition	Hirsutism
Metformin	Hepatic insulin resistance	Obese, IGT or type 2 diabetes
Thiazolidinediones	Adipose tissue and muscle insulin resistance	IGT or type 2 diabetes

of PCOS therapy and cardiovascular outcomes. It also behooves the clinician to remember that the "cure" should not be worse than the disease being treated.

Thiazolidinediones

The thiazolidinediones improve the action of insulin in liver, skeletal muscle, and adipose tissue. Studies in PCOS patients have shown improvement in metabolic phenomena, including insulin levels and sensitivity [109,110]; cardiomyocyte metabolic function [111]; and endothelial function [64]. The thiazolidinediones also lowered vascular inflammation and blood pressure [112], reversing many of the cardiac risk factors associated with diabetes. Ehrmann and coworkers [73] also noted a relative improvement in pancreatic β cell function and a reduction in levels of the prothrombotic factor PAI-1.

In contrast to metformin, which has been used to induce ovulation in infertile women with PCOS and continued into the first trimester of pregnancy, with improved pregnancy outcomes, the thiazolidinediones are contraindicated in pregnancy. They might be considered in women using reliable contraception or preferably in postmenopausal women.

Summary

All of the known risks for cardiovascular disease are increased in women with PCOS. Epidemiologic studies in these patients and their families have revealed a familial predisposition not only to PCOS, but also diabetes, hypertension, and cardiovascular disease. Constructing a prospective longitudinal study with appropriately defined patients and controls, acknowledging previous or ongoing treatments, would be a challenge. Given the importance of cardiovascular disease in women, however, this is a challenge that must be met.

References

[1] Knochenhauer E. Prevalence of the polycystic ovary syndrome in unselected black and white women of the southeastern United States: a prospective study. J Clin Endocrinol Metab 1998;83:3078–82.

[2] Azziz R, Woods KS, Reyna R, et al. The prevalence and features of the polycystic ovary syndrome in an unselected population. J Clin Endocrinol Metab 2004;89:2745–9.

[3] Stein IF, Leventhal M. Amenorrhea associated with bilateral polycystic ovaries. Am J Obstet Gynecol 1935;29:181–91.

[4] Revised 2003 consensus on diagnostic criteria and long-term health risks related to polycystic ovary syndrome (PCOS). Hum Reprod 2004;19:41–7.

[5] Morley JE, Patrick P, Perry HM 3rd. Evaluation of assays available to measure free testosterone. Metabolism 2002;51:554–9.

[6] Carmina E, Chu MC, Longo RA, et al. Phenotypic variation in hyperandrogenic women influences the findings of abnormal metabolic and cardiovascular risk parameters. J Clin Endocrinol Metab 2005;90:2545–9.

[7] Balen AH, Laven JS, Tan SL, et al. Ultrasound assessment of the polycystic ovary: international consensus definitions. Hum Reprod Update 2003;9:505–14.

[8] Ehrmann DA, Barnes RB, Rosenfield RL. Polycystic ovary syndrome as a form of functional ovarian hyperandrogenism due to dysregulation of androgen secretion. Endocr Rev 1995;16:322–53.

[9] Ehrmann DA, Rosenfield RL, Barnes RB, et al. Detection of functional ovarian hyperandrogenism in women with androgen excess. N Engl J Med 1992;327:157–62.

[10] Rosenfield RL. Ovarian and adrenal function in polycystic ovary syndrome. Endocrinol Metab Clin North Am 1999;28:265–93.

[11] Legro RS, Strauss JF. Molecular progress in infertility: polycystic ovary syndrome. Fertil Steril 2002;78:569–76.

[12] Plymate SR, Hoop RC, Jones RE, et al. Regulation of sex hormone-binding globulin production by growth factors. Metabolism 1990;39:967–70.

[13] Silfen ME, Denburg MR, Manibo AM, et al. Early endocrine, metabolic, and sonographic characteristics of polycystic ovary syndrome (PCOS): comparison between nonobese and obese adolescents. J Clin Endocrinol Metab 2003;88:4682–8.

[14] Conway G. Heterogeneity in the polycystic ovary syndrome: clinical, endocrine and ultrasound features in 556 patients. Clin Endocrinol (Oxf) 1989;30:459–70.

[15] Nestler JE, Barlascini CO, Matt DW, et al. Suppression of serum insulin by diazoxide reduces serum testosterone levels in obese women with polycystic ovary syndrome. J Clin Endocrinol Metab 1989;68:1027–32.

[16] Toscano V. Lack of linear relationship between hyperinsulinemia and hyperandrogenism. Clin Endocrinol (Oxf) 1992;36:197–202.

[17] Nelson VL, Qin Kn KN, Rosenfield RL, et al. The biochemical basis for increased testosterone production in theca cells propagated from patients with polycystic ovary syndrome. J Clin Endocrinol Metab 2001;86:5925–33.

[18] Legro RS, Strauss JF. Molecular progress in infertility: polycystic ovary syndrome. Fertil Steril 2002;78:569–76.

[19] Ferriman D, Purdie AW. The inheritance of polycystic ovarian disease and a possible relationship to premature balding. Clin Endocrinol (Oxf) 1979;11:291–300.

[20] Falcone T, Finegood DT, Fantus IG, et al. Androgen response to endogenous insulin secretion during the frequently sampled intravenous glucose tolerance test in normal and hyperandrogenic women. J Clin Endocrinol Metab 1990;71:1653–7.

[21] Rajaniemi HJ, Ronnberg L, Kauppila A, et al. Luteinizing hormone receptors in ovarian follicles of patients with polycystic ovarian disease. J Clin Endocrinol Metab 1980;51:1054–7.

[22] Cataldo NA. Insulin-like growth factor binding proteins: do they play a role in polycystic ovary syndrome? Semin Reprod Endocrinol 1997;15:123–36.

[23] Imse V, Holzapfel G, Hinney B, et al. Comparison of luteinizing hormone pulsatility in the serum of women suffering from polycystic ovarian disease using a bioassay and five different immunoassays. J Clin Endocrinol Metab 1992;74:1053–61.

[24] Azziz R, Ehrmann D, Legro RS, et al. Troglitazone improves ovulation and hirsutism in the polycystic ovary syndrome: a multicenter, double blind, placebo-controlled trial. J Clin Endocrinol Metab 2001;86:1626–32.

[25] Mokdad AH, Ford ES, Bowman BA, et al. Prevalence of obesity, diabetes, and obesity-related health risk factors, 2001. JAMA 2003;289:76–9.

[26] Evans DJ, Hoffmann RG, Kalkhoff RK, et al. Relationship of androgenic activity to body fat topography, fat cell morphology, and metabolic aberrations in premenopausal women. J Clin Endocrinol Metab 1983;57:304–10.

[27] Pasquali R, Casimirri F. The impact of obesity on hyperandrogenism and polycystic ovary syndrome in premenopausal women. Clin Endocrinol (Oxf) 1993;39:1–16.

[28] Bringer J, Lefebvre P, Boulet F, et al. Body composition and regional fat distribution in polycystic ovarian syndrome: relationship to hormonal and metabolic profiles. Ann N Y Acad Sci 1993;687:115–23.

[29] Kirchengast S, Huber J. Body composition characteristics and body fat distribution in lean women with polycystic ovary syndrome. Hum Reprod 2001;16:1255–60.

[30] Douchi T, Ijuin H, Nakamura S, et al. Body fat distribution in women with polycystic ovary syndrome. Obstet Gynecol 1995;86(4 Pt 1):516–9.

[31] Rebuffe-Scrive M, Cullberg G, Lundberg PA, et al. Anthropometric variables and metabolism in polycystic ovarian disease. Horm Metab Res 1989;21:391–7.

[32] Acien P, Quereda F, Matallin P, et al. Insulin, androgens, and obesity in women with and without polycystic ovary syndrome: a heterogeneous group of disorders. Fertil Steril 1999; 72:32–40.

[33] Hollmann M, Runnebaum B, Gerhard I. Effects of weight loss on the hormonal profile in obese, infertile women. Hum Reprod 1996;11:1884–91.

[34] Lefebvre P, Bringer J, Renard E, et al. Influences of weight, body fat patterning and nutrition on the management of PCOS. Hum Reprod 1997;12(Suppl 1):72–81.

[35] Kahn SE, Prigeon RL, McCulloch DK, et al. Quantification of the relationship between insulin sensitivity and beta-cell function in human subjects: evidence for a hyperbolic function. Diabetes 1993;42:1663–72.

[36] Goodarzi MO, Erickson S, Port SC, et al. Relative impact of insulin resistance and obesity on cardiovascular risk factors in polycystic ovary syndrome. Metabolism 2003;52:713–9.

[37] Kiddy DS, Hamilton-Fairley D, Bush A, et al. Improvement in endocrine and ovarian function during dietary treatment of obese women with polycystic ovary syndrome. Clin Endocrinol (Oxf) 1992;36:105–11.

[38] Diamond MP, Grainger D, Diamond MC, et al. Effects of methyltestosterone on insulin secretion and sensitivity in women. J Clin Endocrinol Metab 1998;83:4420–5.

[39] Dunaif A, Green G, Futterweit W, et al. Suppression of hyperandrogenism does not improve peripheral or hepatic insulin resistance in the polycystic ovary syndrome. J Clin Endocrinol Metab 1990;70:699–704.

[40] Venkatesan AM, Dunaif A, Corbould A. Insulin resistance in polycystic ovary syndrome: progress and paradoxes. Recent Prog Horm Res 2001;56:295–308.

[41] Rosenbaum D, Haber RS, Dunaif A. Insulin resistance in polycystic ovary syndrome: decreased expression of GLUT-4 glucose transporters in adipocytes. Am J Physiol 1993; 264(2 Pt 1):E197–202.

[42] Ciaraldi TP, el-Roeiy A, Madar Z, et al. Cellular mechanisms of insulin resistance in polycystic ovarian syndrome. J Clin Endocrinol Metab 1992;75:577–83.

[43] Zhang LH, Rodriguez H, Ohno S, et al. Serine phosphorylation of human P450c17 increases 17,20-lyase activity: implications for adrenarche and the polycystic ovary syndrome. Proc Natl Acad Sci U S A 1995;92:10619–23.

[44] Legro RS, Kunselman AR, Dodson WC, et al. Prevalence and predictors of risk for type 2 diabetes mellitus and impaired glucose tolerance in polycystic ovary syndrome: a prospective, controlled study in 254 affected women. J Clin Endocrinol Metab 1999;84:165–9.

[45] Yilmaz M, Bukan N, Ersoy R, et al. Glucose intolerance, insulin resistance and cardiovascular risk factors in first degree relatives of women with polycystic ovary syndrome. Hum Reprod 2005;20:2414–20.

[46] Kaushal R, Parchure N, Bano G, et al. Insulin resistance and endothelial dysfunction in the brothers of Indian subcontinent Asian women with polycystic ovaries. Clin Endocrinol (Oxf) 2004;60:322–8.

[47] Sam S, Dunaif A. Polycystic ovary syndrome: syndrome XX? Trends Endocrinol Metab 2003;14:365–70.

[48] Apridonidze T, Essah PA, Iuorno MJ, et al. Prevalence and characteristics of the metabolic syndrome in women with polycystic ovary syndrome. J Clin Endocrinol Metab 2005;90: 1929–35.

[49] Dahlgren E, Janson PO, Johansson S, et al. Polycystic ovary syndrome and risk for myocardial infarction: evaluated from a risk factor model based on a prospective population study of women. Acta Obstet Gynecol Scand 1992;71:599–604.

[50] Buggs C, Rosenfield RL. Polycystic ovary syndrome in adolescence. Endocrinol Metab Clin North Am 2005;34:677–705.

[51] Dahlgren E, Johansson S, Lindstedt G, et al. Women with polycystic ovary syndrome wedge resected in 1956 to 1965: a long-term follow-up focusing on natural history and circulating hormones. Fertil Steril 1992;57:505–13.

[52] Reaven G. The metabolic syndrome or the insulin resistance syndrome? Different names, different concepts, and different goals. Endocrinol Metab Clin North Am 2004;33:283–303.

[53] Ehrmann DA, Barnes RB, Rosenfield RL, et al. Prevalence of impaired glucose tolerance and diabetes in women with polycystic ovary syndrome. Diabetes Care 1999;22:141–6.

[54] O'Meara N. Defects in beta-cell function functional ovarian hyperandrogenism. J Clin Endocrinol Metab 1993;76:1241.

[55] Haffner SM, Stern MP, Hazuda HP, et al. Cardiovascular risk factors in confirmed prediabetic individuals: does the clock for coronary heart disease start ticking before the onset of clinical diabetes? JAMA 1990;263:2893–8.

[56] Jeppesen J, Hein HO, Suadicani P, et al. High triglycerides and low HDL cholesterol and blood pressure and risk of ischemic heart disease. Hypertension 2000;36:226–32.

[57] Arslanian SA, Lewy VD, Danadian K. Glucose intolerance in obese adolescents with polycystic ovary syndrome: roles of insulin resistance and beta-cell dysfunction and risk of cardiovascular disease. J Clin Endocrinol Metab 2001;86:66–71.

[58] Rexrode KM, Hennekens CH, Willeh WC, et al. A prospective study of body mass index, weight change, and risk of stroke in women. JAMA 1997;277:1539.

[59] Talbott E, Guzick D, Clerici A, et al. Coronary heart disease risk factors in women with polycystic ovary syndrome. Arterioscler Thromb Vasc Biol 1995;15:821–6.

[60] Kelly CJ, Speirs A, Gould GW, et al. Altered vascular function in young women with polycystic ovary syndrome. J Clin Endocrinol Metab 2002;87:742–6.

[61] Orio F Jr, Palomba S, Cascella T, et al. Early impairment of endothelial structure and function in young normal-weight women with polycystic ovary syndrome. J Clin Endocrinol Metab 2004;89:4588–93.

[62] Paradisi G, Steinberg HO, Hempfling A, et al. Polycystic ovary syndrome is associated with endothelial dysfunction. Circulation 2001;103:1410–5.

[63] Kravariti M, Naka KK, Kalantaridou SN, et al. Predictors of endothelial dysfunction in young women with polycystic ovary syndrome. J Clin Endocrinol Metab 2005;90: 5088–95.

[64] Paradisi G, Steinberg HO, Shepard MK, et al. Troglitazone therapy improves endothelial function to near normal levels in women with polycystic ovary syndrome. J Clin Endocrinol Metab 2003;88:576–80.

[65] Diamanti-Kandarakis E, Alexandraki K, Protogerou A, et al. Metformin administration improves endothelial function in women with polycystic ovary syndrome. Eur J Endocrinol 2005;152:749–56.

[66] Tarkun I, Arslan BC, Canturk Z, et al. Endothelial dysfunction in young women with polycystic ovary syndrome: relationship with insulin resistance and low-grade chronic inflammation. J Clin Endocrinol Metab 2004;89:5592–6.

[67] Diamanti-Kandarakis E, Spina G, Kouli C, et al. Increased endothelin-1 levels in women with polycystic ovary syndrome and the beneficial effect of metformin therapy. J Clin Endocrinol Metab 2001;86:4666–73.

[68] Oliver FJ, de la Rubia G, Feener EP, et al. Stimulation of endothelin-1 gene expression by insulin in endothelial cells. J Biol Chem 1991;266:23251–6.

[69] Meissner MH, Zierler BK, Bergelin RO, et al. Coagulation, fibrinolysis, and recanalization after acute deep venous thrombosis. J Vasc Surg 2002;35:278–85.

[70] Folsom AR. Fibrinolytic factors and atherothrombotic events: epidemiological evidence. Ann Med 2000;32(Suppl 1):85–91.

[71] Dereli D, Ozgen G, Buyukkececi F, et al. Platelet dysfunction in lean women with polycystic ovary syndrome and association with insulin sensitivity. J Clin Endocrinol Metab 2003;88: 2263–8.

[72] Macut D, Micic D, Cvijovic G, et al. Cardiovascular risk in adolescent and young adult obese females with polycystic ovary syndrome (PCOS). J Pediatr Endocrinol Metab 2001;14(Suppl 5):1353–9 [discussion: 1365].

[73] Ehrmann DA, Schneider DJ, Sobel BE, et al. Troglitazone improves defects in insulin action, insulin secretion, ovarian steroidogenesis, and fibrinolysis in women with polycystic ovary syndrome. J Clin Endocrinol Metab 1997;82:2108–16.

[74] Velazquez EM, Mendoza S, Hamer T, et al. Metformin therapy in polycystic ovary syndrome reduces hyperinsulinemia, insulin resistance, hyperandrogenemia, and systolic blood pressure, while facilitating normal menses and pregnancy. Metabolism 1994;43: 647–54.

[75] Benitez R, Sir-Petermann T, Palomino A, et al. [Prevalence of metabolic disorders among family members of patients with polycystic ovary syndrome]. Rev Med Chil 2001;129: 707–12.

[76] Legro RS, Kunselman AR, Dunaif A. Prevalence and predictors of dyslipidemia in women with polycystic ovary syndrome. Am J Med 2001;111:607–13.

[77] Sam S, Legro RS, Bentley-Lewis R, et al. Dyslipidemia and metabolic syndrome in the sisters of women with polycystic ovary syndrome. J Clin Endocrinol Metab 2005;90: 4797–802.

[78] Anderson LA, McTernan PG, Harte AL, et al. The regulation of HSL and LPL expression by DHT and flutamide in human subcutaneous adipose tissue. Diabetes Obes Metab 2002; 4:209–13.

[79] Berg AH, Scherer PE. Adipose tissue, inflammation, and cardiovascular disease. Circ Res 2005;96:939–49.

[80] Carmina E, Orio F, Palomba S, et al. Evidence for altered adipocyte function in polycystic ovary syndrome. Eur J Endocrinol 2005;152:389–94.

[81] Sills ES, Genton MG, Perloe M, et al. Plasma homocysteine, fasting insulin, and androgen patterns among women with polycystic ovaries and infertility. J Obstet Gynaecol Res 2001; 27:163–8.

[82] Clarke R, Daly L, Robinson K, et al. Hyperhomocysteinemia: an independent risk factor for vascular disease. N Engl J Med 1991;324:1149–55.

[83] Tallova J, Býcýkova M, Hill M. Changes of plasma total homocysteine levels during the menstrual cycle. Eur J Clin Invest 1999;129:1041–4.

[84] Yilmaz M, Biri A, Bukan N, et al. Levels of lipoprotein and homocysteine in non-obese and obese patients with polycystic ovary syndrome. Gynecol Endocrinol 2005;20:258–63.

[85] Randeva HS, Lewandowski KC, Drzewoski J, et al. Exercise decreases plasma total homocysteine in overweight young women with polycystic ovary syndrome. J Clin Endocrinol Metab 2002;87:4496–501.

[86] Vrbikova J, Bicikova M, Tallova J, et al. Homocysteine and steroids levels in metformin treated women with polycystic ovary syndrome. Exp Clin Endocrinol Diabetes 2002;110: 74–6.

[87] Ridker P. C-reactive protein and coronary heart disease. N Engl J Med 2004;351:295–8.

[88] Morin-Papunen L, Rautio K, Ruokonen A, et al. Metformin reduces serum C-reactive protein levels in women with polycystic ovary syndrome. J Clin Endocrinol Metab 2003;88: 4649–54.

[89] Rodin DA, Bano G, Bland JM, et al. Polycystic ovaries and associated metabolic abnormalities in Indian subcontinent Asian women. Clin Endocrinol (Oxf) 1998;49:91–9.

[90] Aarabi M. Coronary risk in South Asians: role of ethnicity and blood sugar. Eur J Cardiovasc Prev Rehabil 2004;11:389–93.

[91] Pierpoint T, McKeigue PM, Isaacs AJ, et al. Mortality of women with polycystic ovary syndrome at long-term follow-up. J Clin Epidemiol 1998;51:581–6.

[92] Wild SH. Cardiovascular disease in women with polycystic ovary syndrome at long-term follow-up: a retrospective cohort study. Clin Endocrinol (Oxf) 2000;52:595–600.

[93] Solomon CG, Hu FB, Dunaif A, et al. Menstrual cycle irregularity and risk for future cardiovascular disease. J Clin Endocrinol Metab 2002;87:2013–7.

[94] Rexrode KM, Manson JE, Lee IM, et al. Sex hormone levels and risk of cardiovascular events in postmenopausal women. Circulation 2003;108:1688–93.

[95] Cibula D, Cifkova R, Fanta M, et al. Increased risk of non-insulin dependent diabetes mellitus, arterial hypertension and coronary artery disease in perimenopausal women with a history of the polycystic ovary syndrome. Hum Reprod 2000;15:785–9.

[96] Guzick DS, Talbott EO, Sutton-Tyrell K, et al. Carotid atherosclerosis in women with polycystic ovary syndrome: initial results from a case-control study. Am J Obstet Gynecol 1996; 174:1224.

[97] Talbott EO, Zborowski JV, Boudreaux MY, et al. The relationship between C-reactive protein and carotid intima-media wall thickness in middle-aged women with polycystic ovary syndrome. J Clin Endocrinol Metab 2004;89:6061–7.

[98] Talbott EO, Zborowski JV, Rager JR, et al. Evidence for an association between metabolic cardiovascular syndrome and coronary and aortic calcification among women with polycystic ovary syndrome. J Clin Endocrinol Metab 2004;89:5454–61.

[99] Christian RC, Dumesic DA, Behrenbeck T, et al. Prevalence and predictors of coronary artery calcification in women with polycystic ovary syndrome. J Clin Endocrinol Metab 2003;88:2562–8.

[100] Orio F Jr, Palomba S, Spinelli L, et al. The cardiovascular risk of young women with polycystic ovary syndrome: an observational, analytical, prospective case-control study. J Clin Endocrinol Metab 2004;89:3696–701.

[101] Yarali H, Yildirir A, Aybar F, et al. Diastolic dysfunction and increased serum homocysteine concentrations may contribute to increased cardiovascular risk in patients with polycystic ovary syndrome. Fertil Steril 2001;76:511–6.

[102] Tiras MB, Yalcin R, Noyan V, et al. Alterations in cardiac flow parameters in patients with polycystic ovarian syndrome. Hum Reprod 1999;14:1949–52.

[103] Wild RA, Grubb B, Hartz A, et al. Clinical signs of androgen excess as risk factors for coronary artery disease. Fertil Steril 1990;54:255–9.

[104] Birdsall MA, Farquhar CM, White HD. Association between polycystic ovaries and extent of coronary artery disease in women having cardiac catheterization. Ann Intern Med 1997; 126:32–5.

[105] Legro RS. Polycystic ovary syndrome and cardiovascular disease: a premature association? Endocr Rev 2003;24:302–12.

[106] Knowler WC, Barrett-Connor E, Fowler SE, et al. Reduction in the incidence of type 2 diabetes with lifestyle intervention or metformin. N Engl J Med 2002;346:393–403.

[107] Penna IA. Acarbose in obese patients with polycystic ovarian syndrome: a double-blind, randomized, placebo-controlled study. Hum Reprod 2005;20:2396–401.

[108] Kilicdag EB, Bagis T, Zeyneloglu HB, et al. Homocysteine levels in women with polycystic ovary syndrome treated with metformin versus rosiglitazone: a randomized study. Hum Reprod 2005;20:894–9.

[109] Ghazeeri G, Kutteh WH, Bryer-Ash M, et al. Effect of rosiglitazone on spontaneous and clomiphene citrate-induced ovulation in women with polycystic ovary syndrome. Fertil Steril 2003;79:562–6.

[110] Azziz R, Ehrmann DA, Legro RS, et al. Troglitazone decreases adrenal androgen levels in women with polycystic ovary syndrome. Fertil Steril 2003;79:932–7.

[111] Sidell RJ, Cole MA, Draper NJ, et al. Thiazolidinedione treatment normalizes insulin resistance and ischemic injury in the Zucker fatty rat heart. Diabetes 2002;51:1110–7.
[112] Lord JM, Flight IH, Norman RJ. Insulin-sensitising drugs (metformin, troglitazone, rosiglitazone, pioglitazone, D-chiro-inositol) for polycystic ovary syndrome. Cochrane Database Syst Rev 2003;3:CD003053.

ELSEVIER
SAUNDERS

Endocrinol Metab Clin N Am
35 (2006) 633–649

ENDOCRINOLOGY
AND METABOLISM
CLINICS
OF NORTH AMERICA

Ethnicity and Diabetic Heart Disease

Jatin K. Dave, MD, MPH[a], Vikram V. Kamdar, MD[b],*

[a]Harvard Medical School, Division of Aging, Brigham and Women's Hospital,
1620 Tremont Street, Boston, MA 02120, USA
[b]Division of Endocrinology, Diabetes, and Hypertension, David Geffen School
of Medicine at UCLA, Santa Monica UCLA Medical Center,
1801 Wilshire Boulevard, Santa Monica, CA 90403, USA

Of the more than 20 million adults in the United States with diabetes, about 7 million have diabetic heart disease (DHD), which translates into an approximately 30% prevalence of DHD [1]. Although there are many definitions of DHD [2,3], for the purpose of this discussion, DHD is defined as heart disease, including coronary artery disease (CAD) and heart failure, in patients with diabetes mellitus (DM). DHD is a major public health problem around the globe because of the rising prevalence of diabesity. Diabetes is the single most important risk factor for CAD; diabetes confers a risk equivalent to that associated with already having had a CAD-related event. CAD is responsible for causing 55% of deaths in adults with diabetes [4,5]. Diabetes is also an independent predictor of poor outcome in patients with heart disease [6]. Prevention and management of diabetes is of paramount importance for continued cardiovascular risk reduction as most other CAD risk factors have declined in recent decades. Over the past 30 years, for example, deaths from CAD declined by 27% in nondiabetic women but increased by 23% in diabetic women [7,8]. Thus diabetes is increasingly recognized as not only a metabolic disorder but also a vascular disorder [9].

DHD is a complex disease caused by the interplay between genetic and environmental factors, influenced by ethnicity. Considering the increasing ethnic diversity found in the United States, and since as much as 35% of the increase in diabetes incidence in the United States can be attributed to minority population increases [10], it is imperative that we unravel these complex interactions to better understand the mechanisms involved in the development of CAD to provide more effective, culturally sensitive prevention and treatment strategies.

---

* Corresponding author.
E-mail address: VKamdar@mednet.ucla.edu (V.V. Kamdar).

0889-8529/06/$ - see front matter © 2006 Elsevier Inc. All rights reserved.
doi:10.1016/j.ecl.2006.06.004

Despite the debate over the use of ethnicity in medicine, it remains a powerful predictor of health and is of increasing importance in the United States because of the growth in minority ethnic populations [11,12]. Recognizing the importance and potential for misuse, many journals have recently published useful guidelines on the use of race and ethnicity in articles [13]. The American Diabetic Association has also endorsed race/ethnicity as a risk factor for Type 2 diabetes mellitus. An ethnicity-based approach to diabetes is also important because of the observed disparities in the prevalence of DM and its complications (such as end-stage renal disease) with a greater burden of diabetes in minority populations [14,15]. To eliminate variations in outcomes, we need to understand the variations and target our efforts at those at greatest risk for disabling complications.

Ethnicity is an especially useful construct (compared with race) for DHD since it combines social and cultural values (ie, effects of lifestyle) in addition to biologic predispositions. Impact on health can be potentially caused via ethnicity-based variations in genetic, socioeconomic, lifestyle, and treatment factors. Awareness of ethnicity-specific information about DHD will help provide better patient-centered, evidence-based and culturally competent care. Such patient-centered cultural awareness is of higher importance now as a result of increasing globalization (that is progressively greater influence of worldwide economic, social, and cultural processes over local trends) and migration.

CAD is the leading cause of death and disability-adjusted life year losses around the globe [16]. Although CAD-associated deaths in developed countries have declined in recent years, they have been dramatically increasing in developing countries [17] so that now as much as 80% of global CAD burden is reported in developing countries [18]. The most significant factor contributing to this shift is the increased prevalence of obesity, metabolic syndrome, and diabetes in developing countries as a result of increasing urbanization, industrialization, and increasing energy consumption in the form of concentrated calories and fat [17]. These changes have also resulted in increased salt consumption and potential psychological stress from acculturation and migration. There is a pressing need to develop and implement strategies for global prevention of obesity, diabetes, and DHD. Greater understanding of ethnicity-based variations may provide building blocks for designing such strategies.

In this article we review the literature focusing on ethnic variations and similarities in prevalence, risk factors, and management of DHD. Since approximately 90% to 95% of diabetic Americans have Type 2 diabetes, this review focuses on DHD in patients with this form of disease [1]. Each ethnicity represents a diverse group of populations, making it impossible to describe all groups in detail. In addition, despite the growth of literature in the field of diabetes and heart disease, quality data for ethnicity and heart disease in patients with diabetes are scant. Therefore, we attempt to provide an overview of information on selected ethnic groups living in the developed countries with an in-depth description in Asian Indians as an example to highlight the importance of ethnicity in management of DHD. We focus on Asian Indians since they are one of the best-studied ethnic groups and currently have the highest prevalence of diabetes in the world, with more than 30 million patients in India [19]. Asian Indians also have the highest predicted increase in prevalence of diabetes by 2030 owing to epidemiologic transition, a theory that predicts relatively constant changes in disease patterns during the development of societies [20]. A unique predisposition to insulin resistance in native and immigrant Asian Indians has raised several useful questions on mechanism of CAD, and many studies are ongoing to answer these questions.

Epidemiology of diabetic heart disease by ethnicity

Prevalence and incidence

Understanding the relationship between obesity, metabolic syndrome, diabetes, and DHD is essential for more effective prevention and treatment of DHD, since up to 54% of patients with DM are obese [21] and metabolic syndrome accounts for up to half of new-onset diabetes cases and one third of CAD risk [22]. Ethnic prevalences of obesity, metabolic syndrome, diabetes, and DHD are shown in Table 1 to illustrate the continuum of interethnic variations from obesity to DHD [23]. However, note that Table 1 data for American Indians [24] and Asian Indians, included for the sake of completion, were not drawn from national representative surveys, limiting comparisons among these data and those from the other ethnic groups owing to potential differences in study design. As shown in this table, there are remarkably different risks for the development of metabolic syndrome among ethnic groups and genders within ethnic groups, which do not appear to correlate well with the corresponding prevalence of obesity. Hispanic American women have markedly more metabolic syndrome than African American women, despite having a lower prevalence of obesity, while African American men have a much lower risk of metabolic syndrome than Hispanic American or non-Hispanic white men despite having a similar risk of obesity. American Indians have by far the worst prevalence of metabolic syndrome and diabetes, despite obesity rates that are not appreciably different than those found in other ethnic groups. A better understanding of this differential risk for metabolic syndrome by ethnicity is of critical importance [25].

A trend in the prevalence of diabetes by ethnicity over the past 2 decades (Fig. 1) shows a recent increase in the prevalence of diabetes in all ethnic groups except Hispanic American women, although both African American and Hispanic American men and women still demonstrate substantially higher prevalence than white men and women. The incidence of diabetes in 1998 to 2000 among adults was estimated at 9.5, 9.0, 8.5, 8.0, and 5.0 per 1000 in Native-, African-, Hispanic-, Asian-, and Caucasian- Americans,

Table 1
Prevalence of obesity, metabolic syndrome, diabetes, and diabetic heart disease in US adults by ethnicity (%)

Ethnicity	Obesity [74]		Metabolic syndrome† [75]		Diabetes‡ [21]		DHD [76]	
	Men	Women	Men	Women	Men	Women	Men	Women
Non-Hispanic White	27.3 (1.82)	30.1 (2.1)	24.8 (1.4)	22.8 (1.1)	2.9–8.4	2.5–7.8	38.7	30.7
African American	28.1 (2.27)	49.7 (2.79)	16.4 (1.1)	25.7 (1.3)	8.5	12.1	31.3	28.9
Hispanic/Mexican American	28.9 (2.25)	39.7 (3.65)	28.3 (1.8)	35.6 (1.5)	7.2–16.7	4.5–19	29.9	23.7
Chinese American			15.9	7.1				
All	27.5 (1.61)	33.4 (3.65)	24 (1.1)	23.4 (0.9)			33.3*	27.8*
South Asians§ [54]			23.4	28.3				
American Indian§,|| [25]	38.5 (2.84)	29.4 (2.53)	55.2		20			13.2

* Estimate based on Non-Hispanic white, African- and Hispanic/Mexican-American data only.
† ATP III definition, using NHANES III–1988–1994.
‡ Range variations due to data from different sources.
§ Study designs are different from other groups.
|| Data available only in for subjects age 45–74 years.

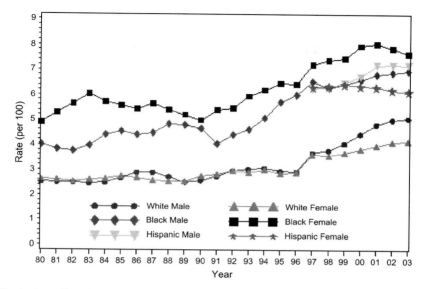

Fig. 1. Age-adjusted prevalence of diagnosed diabetes by race/ethnicity and sex, United States, 1980–2003 (*From* Centers for Disease Control Diabetes Public Health Resource. Available at: http://www.cdc.gov/diabetes/statistics/prev/national/figraceethsex.htm).

respectively [26]. The risk ratios for diabetes in Native-, African-, Hispanic- and Asian- Americans were 2.2, 1.8, 1.7, 1.5, and 1.5, respectively, when compared with Caucasian Americans [1,27]. Thus non-Caucasian ethnic groups in the United States, in general, have both a higher prevalence and incidence of diabetes mellitus than Caucasians, emphasizing the importance of ethnicity-sensitive prevention and management strategies.

To be or not to be: a paradox of higher diabetes mellitus and lower coronary artery disease risk

It remains controversial whether or not, despite increased risk of diabetes, African, Hispanic, and Native Americans have paradoxically lower CAD prevalence. Explanations used to argue against the existence of a paradox include variations in study design with ethnic misclassification, differential ascertainment of deaths, and variable adjustment of socioeconomic status [28]. Those who favor the paradox suggest an insulin-sensitive variant of diabetes in African Americans, healthy migrant effects in Hispanic Americans, and effect modification by gender in Native Americans [29]. Recent radiological studies have shown lower prevalence of coronary artery calcification and obstructive coronary disease in Hispanic, African, and Asian Americans, supporting the paradox [30–32]. Regardless of the presence or absence of the paradox, ie, even if we assume the lower relative risk of CAD, the absolute risk of DHD in many ethnic populations, such as Hispanic Americans, may be increasing because of the rising prevalence of obesity-associated diabetes.

Overview of epidemiology of diabetic heart disease by ethnicity

The majority of the literature on DHD in the United States focuses on Caucasians (also described as white or non-Hispanic), who constitute about 70% of the total population at present, but who are projected to represent only about 50% by 2050 [33]. Caucasians are commonly of European descent and generally have a higher prevalence of dyslipidemia than other populations. Over the past 5 decades, the prevalence of obesity, metabolic syndrome, and diabetes has continued to increase in Caucasians [34]. The most recent estimate of diabetes prevalence in Caucasians is 8.7%, translating into 1.31 million Caucasians in the United States with diabetes.

African Americans represent about 13% of the US population and are projected to increase to 15% of the total population by 2050. Hypertension appears to be a stronger risk factor for CAD than diabetes in African Americans than non-Hispanic whites [35]. African Americans have a higher prevalence of obesity, diabetes, and hypertension but relatively healthy lipid profiles and a relatively low prevalence of metabolic syndrome, especially among men. African Americans have twice the diabetes prevalence of Caucasians [36], but have slightly lower relative CAD risk than non-Hispanic whites. While the reasons for this disparity are not clear, studies suggest that many African Americans have an insulin-sensitive form of diabetes, which may contribute to their risk reduction [28]. Coronary artery calcium and subclinical atherosclerosis is also lower in African Americans than in Caucasians with or without DM [30,37]. A recent study comparing process and outcome measures of diabetes care across ethnicity showed poorer control of diabetes and hypertension in African Americans than in Caucasian or Hispanic Americans [38].

Hispanic Americans compose about 13.7% of the total US population, a percentage that is projected to double by 2050. Hispanic Americans have a higher prevalence of obesity, metabolic syndrome, and diabetes than non-Hispanic whites, but it remains questionable whether they also have a higher prevalence of coronary artery disease. Among Hispanic populations, Mexican Americans have the highest and Cuban Americans have the lowest prevalence of diabetes, however all three subgroups (Mexican and Cuban American and Puerto Rican) have a higher prevalence of diabetes than non-Hispanic Caucasians [39]. Among Hispanic Americans, the prevalence of diabetes is estimated at about 9.5%, affecting 2.5 million adults [1]. Hispanic patients with diabetes also generally have poorer control of their hypertension than Caucasian patients, further increasing their risk for CAD [38].

Native Americans constitute about 1.5% of the total US population and have the highest prevalence of DM in the United States. Approximately 12.8% of this population, or more than 99 500 Native Americans, have diabetes [1]. Although earlier studies showed a lower prevalence of heart disease among Native Americans with DM than non-Hispanic whites [40], the most recent data from the Strong Heart Study show a higher prevalence of CAD in diabetic Native Americans [41].

Asian Americans currently represent about 4% of the total US population and are projected to double to 8% of the total population by 2050. This ethnicity includes at least 10 diverse subgroups, although 5 ethnic groups (Chinese [24%], Filipino [18%], Asian Indians [16%], Vietnamese [11%], and Korean [10%]) constitute more than two thirds of this population. Japanese, Cambodian, Hmong, Laotian, Pakistani, and Thai compose the remainder of this group. Because of their significantly increased risk for DHD, we present data on South Asians (Indians, Pakistanis, and Bangladeshis) in greater detail below to highlight the significance of ethnicity in DHD. South Asians have a higher prevalence of DM and metabolic syndrome than other Asian Americans, despite a significantly lower prevalence of obesity and cigarette smoking. According to one study, the risk of DM with weight gain was 1.6 times higher in South Asians than in Caucasians. The exact reasons for this paradoxical increase in the risk of DM are not known. Studies have shown increased insulin resistance in Indian subjects even without overt obesity [42,43]. Studies of interethnic variations are needed, since improved understanding of the etiology of increased insulin resistance in this population, for example, should not only help better manage DM in South Asians but may also provide general insight into the mechanisms of DM [44].

Impact of ethnicity on coronary artery disease risk factors

The goal of an ethnicity-based approach to DHD prevention is to identify high-risk patients for more aggressive (earlier and more frequent) screening for DM and its associated metabolic disorders and to achieve risk reduction via lifestyle modifications and aggressive management of associated risk factors in appropriate patients. Improved understanding of ethnic variations in predisposing mechanisms to DHD will help us develop individualized strategies to prevent DHD (Table 2).

More than 300 risk factors have been associated with coronary artery disease and these can be divided into (1) major/conventional risk factors with high prevalence, independent effect on risk, and reduced risk of outcome with treatment and (2) minor/novel risk factors without such characteristics.

Table 2

Comparison of traditional cardiovascular risk factors in patients with diabetes mellitus by ethnicity [77–79]

Ethnicity	HTN	HCH	Smoking
Caucasian	62.8	54.8	17.2
African American	72.6	54.2	20.6
Hispanic	54.7	51.8	13.1
Asian Americans	49.7	49.3	14
American Indian	59.9	50.7	31.2

Abbreviations: DM, diabetes mellitus; HTN, hypertension; HCH, hypercholesteremia.

Assessment of the major risk factors, such as hypertension, hypercholesterolemia, and smoking in patients with DM is of critical importance since these risk factors act synergistically with DM. Glycemic control should also be carefully monitored as it is known to be another important CAD risk factor.

Recently, researchers have studied whether the interethnic variations in risk for DHD can be explained by the differences in risk factors. Although the prevalence of conventional risk factors varies by ethnicity, these differences only partly explain the interethnic variability in the CAD risk. Caucasians have a higher prevalence of hypercholesterolemia, while African Americans have a higher prevalence of hypertension and smoking. Asian Americans have a lower prevalence of all three of these traditional cardiovascular risk factors despite their disproportionately high CAD risk. The limitations of conventional risk factors to explain such variability have led to the emergence of many novel cardiovascular risk factors.

Interest in novel CAD risk factors initially stemmed from the notion that fewer than 50% of patients with CAD have traditional risk factors, although more recent studies have refuted this conclusion [45,46]. However, the high prevalence of CAD risk factors in those without CAD and the inability of conventional risk factors to fully explain the excess risk in certain ethnic populations have led to the emergence of many novel risk factors to further refine the CAD risk assessment. These nontraditional risk factors support inflammation as the primary mechanism for the development of DHD. Studies on novel risk factors are especially needed in certain ethnic population such as South Asians, who have a high prevalence of CAD risk despite low prevalence of conventional risk factors. Nontraditional risk factors can be divided into three groups: (1) novel lipid markers (eg, lipoprotein [a], triglycerides, Apolipoprotein B, and small dense low-density lipoprotein [LDL]), (2) inflammatory markers (eg, C-reactive protein [CRP], leukocyte count, and homocysteine), and (3) prothrombotic markers (eg, plasminogen activator inhibitor-1 [PAI-1], fibrinogen, von Willebrand factor, and factor VIII activity).

Little comparative information across ethnic groups is available about any possible relationship between novel risk factors for CAD in patients with diabetes. We found no study comparing novel risk factors across multiple ethnicities in patients with diabetes. Despite multiple prospective studies showing that CRP is an independent predictor of vascular risk, rigorous prospective data in minority groups with diabetes are nonexistent. We found two studies evaluating CRP in patients with diabetes; neither reported data on ethnicity [47,48]. Thus, the current data on novel risk factors in ethnic populations with diabetes require extrapolation to extract data from studies on Caucasians or from studies on patients without diabetes.

The Atherosclerosis Risk in Communities (ARIC) study, which enrolled 1676 diabetic subjects, showed that levels of albumin, fibrinogen, and von Willebrand factor; factor VIII activity; and leukocyte count were associated with the incidence of coronary heart disease in diabetic subjects, independent of traditional risk factors. The authors did not report the results by ethnicity [49].

Other studies of novel risk factors in ethnic populations do not report results in patients with diabetes separately. The Study of Health Assessment and Risk In Ethnic groups (SHARE) from Canada showed higher CRP levels among aboriginal (native) Canadians and South Asians compared with Chinese and Europeans [50]. These differences diminished but persisted after adjustment for metabolic risk factors. Higher CRP levels were also seen in South Asian women compared with European women in a small study from London [51]. Another study from Canada that examined CAD risk in Europeans, Chinese, and South Asians, including patients with diabetes (but which did not report results from patients with diabetes separately), reported greater abnormalities in prothrombotic markers such as fibrinogen, PAI-1 lipoprotein (a) and homocysteine in South Asians than in the other groups [52]. In addition, South Asians had lower levels of atherosclerosis, as measured by carotid intima media thickness (IMT), but a paradoxically higher CAD event rate. Elevations in nontraditional risk factors in the South Asian population suggest the possibility of a proinflammatory or prothrombotic state that could contribute to their CAD risk, while their disproportional high CAD event rate for their atherosclerotic plaque burden also suggests that increased destabilization of vulnerable atherosclerotic plaque may contribute to the CAD risk of this group.

Lipoprotein (a) levels are thought to be genetically determined, and are 2 to 3 times higher in African Americans than in Caucasians. South Asians also usually have higher levels than Caucasians. However, there is no demonstrated correlation between lipoprotein (a) levels and increased cardiovascular disease risk in these minority ethnic populations [53]. Plasma homocysteine levels are higher in premenopausal African American woman and South Asians than Caucasians. These levels have been attributed to the habit of thoroughly cooking the vegetables consumed by these two ethnic groups, reducing their dietary folic acid and vitamin B12 intake and consequently increasing their plasma homocysteine levels.

Overview of epidemiology in South Asians with special emphasis on Asian Indians

South Asia is a subregion of Asia, usually considered to comprise the modern countries of Bangladesh, Bhutan, India, Nepal, Pakistan, and Sri Lanka. South Asians account for 25% of deaths related to CAD worldwide [54]. Coronary heart disease is likely to cause for around 33.5% of total deaths by the year 2015 and would replace infectious disease as a number one killer in India [55]. The World Health Organization predicts that by 2010, South Asian Indian patients will constitute 60% of the world's cardiac patients, which translates into more than 100 million South Asian Indians with CAD [18,56]. Based on current trends, India will be the largest single contributor to global coronary artery disease mortality. The prevalence of diabetes in migrant populations from India living in the United States, the United Kingdom, and South Africa is as high as 16% [57,58], and CAD is 1.5 to 10 times more common in Asian Indians compared with the general population of the host country. South Asian migrants also have higher CAD mortality than the local populations [59].

In the United States, 4.1% of the population is of Asian descent, 16% of whom are of South Asian ancestry and South Asians are the fastest growing population in the United States [54]. The data on South Asians living in the United States is limited but the existing data support a higher prevalence of CAD and increased CAD mortality than the non-Hispanic white population. For example, the prevalence of CAD in South Asian Indian physicians is 3 to 4 times higher than that of the non-Hispanic white physician population of the United States [60].

Asian Indians, like many other populations, have been shown to have normal diabetes progression, starting with normal glucose tolerance, but developing insulin resistance and compensatory hyperinsulinemia, before progressing to impaired glucose tolerance and overt diabetes. The development of diabetes is closely associated with the presence of obesity. The relative contribution of insulin secretion and insulin resistance appears to differ by ethnicity. As described, African Americans have an insulin-sensitive variant of diabetes; in contrast, Asian Indians have higher insulin resistance.

Risk factors for coronary artery disease in South Asian Indians

Traditional risk factors

In India the prevalence of obesity (body mass index [BMI] $> 30/kg/m^2$) is 2% to 15% in urban Indians versus 0% to 6% in rural populations. However, the prevalence is highest in migrant South Asian Indian populations [54,61]. South Asian Indians have a higher prevalence of body fat in relation to BMI and lower fat-free mass compared with Caucasians and African Americans [62]. The prevalence of abdominal obesity is 9% to 52% of South Asian Indians, and thicker skin folds are noted in South Asian Indians with normal weight [54,55].

South Asian Indians (both native and immigrant population) also have a higher prevalence of glucose intolerance, abdominal obesity, hyperinsulinemia, and hypertriglyceridemia compared with Caucasians [63]. The prevalence of metabolic syndrome in South Asians living in the United Kingdom varies from 5% to 50% of the population depending on the definition of metabolic syndrome (ie, National Cholesterol Education Program guidelines, World Health Organization guidelines, or modified guidelines for the Asian population) [54]. Overall, the prevalence of insulin-resistance syndrome in Asian Indians was higher than in other ethnic groups in various studies. Insulin resistance in Asian Indians manifests early in life, and hyperinsulinemia has been detected in umbilical cords, postpubertal children, and young adults [54]. Healthy sons of Asian Indians with angiographically proven CAD also had a higher magnitude of hyperinsulinemia than did sons of white patients with CAD [54].

The prevalence of diabetes is 4 to 5 times higher (19% versus 4%) in South Asians compared with Caucasians. The prevalence of smoking is variable in South Asian men coming from various South Asian countries, but is very low among females. Low physical activity is a very common finding among the South Asian population and appears to be a significant risk factor for CAD, particularly in immigrant South Asians [55,61]. Paradoxically, low levels of total cholesterol are noted in South Asian patients with CAD. But there is a higher prevalence of high triglycerides and low HDL among the South Asian population, and it is associated with increased cardiovascular risk [54,61]. The presence of high levels of dense LDL is now well documented in South Asians. Lipoprotein (a) is an important novel risk factor and is higher in South Asian Indians than in the Caucasians reported in studies from the United States, the United Kingdom, and India [55,61]. An additional risk factor of increased apoB is found in one third of Asian Indian men [61]. In South Asians, it is not the hypercholesterolemia, but the above-described dyslipidemia that results in a risk of CAD [55,61].

Nontraditional risk factors

South Asians are known to have increased plasma levels of proinflammatory markers (eg, CRP, PAI-1, fibrinogen, homocysteine, and proinflammatory cytokines) [54,55,61,62,] and impaired flow-mediated endothelium-dependent vascular dilatation (endothelial dysfunction) [64].

Unique risk factors

Several studies have reported the low dietary intake and low plasma levels of Omega 3 polyunsaturated fatty acids in lacto-vegetarian South Asian Indians. The prevalence of hyperhomocysteinemia is reported to be higher among South Asians than Caucasians and may be related to cooking habits for dietary vegetables that destroy their folic acid and vitamin B12 content. Increased consumption of coconuts and coconut and palm oils (high in saturated fat) are also implicated in CAD in South Asians. Extensive use of ghee (clarified butter) and partially hydrogenated vegetable oils with a higher content of trans fatty acids adds to the CAD risk [55,61]. Analysis of ghee has revealed high levels of cholesterol oxides, not found in ordinary butter, which are more atherogenic than pure cholesterol in animal studies. The concept that South Asians have smaller coronary vessels has been refuted in recent literature [61].

Impact of ethnicity on management of diabetic heart disease

Ethnicity-based strategies for CAD prevention have been shown to be more effective than generic strategies [65]. Ethnicity-based CAD prevention strategies have implications both for population-based prevention approaches and the management of individual patient care.

Population-based strategies and policy implications

Many studies have documented ethnicity-based variations in quality of care, including variations in screening, glycemic control, and treatment of risk factors [66–70]. As stated in the conclusion of a recent review, "Although no generalizations can be made for all ethnic groups in all regions for all kinds of complications, the results do implicate the importance of quality of care in striving for equal health outcomes among ethnic minorities" [71]. Improvement in overall quality of care has shown to reduce ethnicity-based variations. Several measures could reduce the ethnicity-based disparities in DHD. They include health care policy designed to reduce the variability in ethnicity-based discrepancies to access to care; improved cultural competence of providers, which in turn will improve trust in the health care system; increased opportunities for a healthy diet and exercise; improved educational resources; and access to affordable pharmacotherapy.

Ethnicity-based programs designed to reduce the common barriers that have been identified among a particular ethnic group have been shown to have greater impact than usual care. The intervention group had modest improvement in blood pressure and cholesterol control [65].

Individual-based strategies

It is important to be aware of ethnicity-based cultural values and their implications for management of patient lifestyle changes (reduced saturated and trans fat intake, increased physical activity and weight loss), glycemic control, blood pressure control, and aggressive treatment of other cardiovascular risk factors (aspirin therapy, smoking cessation, and so forth). The South Asians and certain Pacific Islanders are using highly saturated fatty acids in the forms of coconut and palm oil, which should be discouraged, and the clarified butter, ie, ghee, used by the South Asian Indian should also be discouraged [61]. The encouragement for diet with high protein, complex carbohydrates, and lots of fiber does have beneficial effects to improve diabetic dyslipidemia and insulin sensitivity in ethnic groups predisposed to diabesity [62]. The avoidance of overcooking of the vegetables by certain ethnic populations can be a part of the health education of that group.

Many patients with DM fail to receive appropriate screening for risk factors and treatment to achieve the desired goals. Such undertreatment is more common in many ethnic populations. Unfortunately, some of these same populations are also at higher risk of diabetes-related complications and thus could have greater absolute risk reduction if properly screened and treated. Awareness of ethnicity-based variations in prevalence of insulin resistance, propensity for a prothrombogenic environment, and differential cutoffs may improve risk assessment. Current data on such ethnicity-based modifications of national guidelines are nonexistent, and more data are needed to justify ethnicity-based screening and treatment thresholds.

There is also a need for future research on the effect of ethnicity on development and maintenance of health-promoting behaviors. The one-size-fits-all approach may not be appropriate in multiethnic populations because of different cultural beliefs and life experiences of individuals of different ethnicities. A paucity of research on factors related to health-promoting behaviors in ethnic minorities should be noted and such social research should be funded.

Obesity contributes to DHD both as a risk factor for DM and CAD and as a risk factor for hypertension and hyperlipidemia causing the clustering of other cardiovascular risk factors as in the case with metabolic syndrome. Ethnicity modifies obesity-associated cardiovascular risk. African Americans are at increased risk for obesity-associated hypertension, and Hispanic Americans have a higher risk of obesity-associated diabetes [72]. While counseling patients, it is important to ask questions to better understand the patient's values and cultural background, which may increase acceptance and compliance. Thus, prevention efforts should be focused on the ethnicity-based prevalence of risk factors and values.

Future directions in ethnicity and diabetic heart disease

There is a need for ethnicity-specific data; both conventional as well as novel risk factors. The Multi-Ethnic Study of Atherosclerosis is a multisite study of subclinical cardiovascular disease in four ethnic populations: Caucasians, African Americans, Hispanic Americans, and Asian Americans (of Chinese descent) [30]. Initial results from the study indicate differences in pathophysiology of coronary heart disease by ethnicity. Future studies should assess the risk of DHD based on ethnicity to determine whether significant differences may support lower thresholds for certain high-risk ethnicities. Such studies will help improve our understanding of etiology by allowing us to compare the relative contribution of genetic predisposition compared with lifestyle factors.

Admixture mapping may allow us to identify defects in gene flow that have been identified recently in two populations. This technique was used in African-American and Hispanic American populations [73].

Summary

Ethnicity is a complex yet important construct and an independent risk factor for DHD with paramount clinical significance. Clinicians should try to better understand the role of ethnicity through more questions. The risk of DHD is modified by ethnicity, and its management may require a culturally sensitive individualized approach. Findings from Caucasian populations cannot be fully extrapolated to other ethnic groups, thereby emphasizing the importance of future research with ethnicity-specific data. Clinicians should be aware of an ethnicity-based threshold for obesity. Available limited data support the interaction between genetic predisposition, environmental risk, and lifestyle choices and disparities based on ethnicity as the likely cause for ethnic variations in DHD.

References

[1] McCarron P, Davey Smith G. Commentary: Incubation of coronary heart disease–recent developments. Int J Epidemiol 2005;34(2):248–50.

[2] Timmis AD. Diabetic heart disease: clinical considerations. Heart 2001;85(4):463–9.

[3] Marwick TH. Diabetic heart disease. Heart 2006;92(3):296–300.

[4] Whiteley L, Padmanabhan S, Hole D, et al. Should diabetes be considered a coronary heart disease risk equivalent? Results from 25 years of follow-up in the Renfrew and Paisley Survey. Diabetes Care 2005;28(7):1588–93.

[5] Lotufo PA, Gaziano JM, Chae CU, et al. Diabetes and all-cause and coronary heart disease mortality among US male physicians. Arch Intern Med 2001;161(2):242–7.

[6] Almdal T, Scharling H, Jensen JS, et al. The independent effect of type 2 diabetes mellitus on ischemic heart disease, stroke, and death: a population-based study of 13 000 men and women with 20 years of follow-up. Arch Intern Med 2004;164(13):1422–6.

[7] Gregg EW, Cheng YJ, Cadwell BL, et al. Secular trends in cardiovascular disease risk factors according to body mass index in US adults. JAMA 2005;293(15):1868–74.

[8] Gu K, Cowie CC, Harris MI. Diabetes and decline in heart disease mortality in US adults. JAMA 1999;281(14):1291–7.

[9] Deedwania P. Therapeutic strategies in diabetes and cardiovascular disease. Cardiol Clin 2005;23(2):xi–xii.

[10] Rao SV, Mcguire DK. Epidemiology of diabetes mellitus and cardiovascular disease. In: Marso SP, Stern DM, editors. Diabetes and cardiovascaular disease: integrating science and clinical medicine. Philadelphia: Lippincott Williams Wilkins; 2004. p. 156.

[11] Burchard EG, Ziv E, Coyle N, et al. The importance of race and ethnic background in biomedical research and clinical practice. N Engl J Med 2003;348(12):1170–5.

[12] Nickens HW. A compelling research agenda. Ann Intern Med 1996;125(3):237–9.

[13] Kaplan JB, Bennett T. Use of race and ethnicity in biomedical publication. JAMA 2003; 289(20):2709–16.

[14] Narayan KMV, Boyle JP, Thompson TJ, et al. Lifetime risk for diabetes mellitus in the United States. JAMA 2003;290(14):1884–90.

[15] Detrano R. The ethnic-specific natureof mechanisms forcoronary heart disease. J Am Coll Cardiol 2003;41(1):45–6.

[16] Roglic G, Unwin N, Bennett PH, et al. The burden of mortality attributable to diabetes: realistic estimates for the year 2000. Diabetes Care 2005;28(9):2130–5.

[17] Reddy KS, Yusuf S. Emerging epidemic of cardiovascular disease in developing countries. Circulation 1998;97(6):596–601.

[18] Gaziano TA. Cardiovascular disease in the developing world and its cost-effective management. Circulation 2005;112(23):3547–53.

[19] Wild S, Roglic G, Green A, et al. Global prevalence of diabetes: estimates for the year 2000 and projections for 2030. Diabetes Care 2004;27(5):1047–53.

[20] Omran AR. The epidemiologic transition: a theory of the epidemiology of population change. Milbank Q 2005;83(4):731–57.

[21] Carter JS, Pugh JA, Monterrosa A. Non-insulin-dependent diabetes mellitus in minorities in the United States. Ann Intern Med 1996;125(3):221–32.

[22] Prevalence of overweight and obesity among adults with diagnosed diabetes–United States, 1988,–1994 and 1999,–2002. JAMA 2005;293(5):546–7.

[23] Wilson PWF, D'Agostino RB, Parise H, et al. Metabolic syndrome as a precursor of cardiovascular disease and type 2 diabetes mellitus. Circulation 2005;112(20):3066–72.

[24] Ford ES, Giles WH, Dietz WH. Prevalence of the metabolic syndrome among US adults: findings from the Third National Health and Nutrition Examination Survey 10.1001/jama.287.3.356. JAMA 2002;287(3):356–9.

[25] Resnick HE. Metabolic syndrome in American Indians. Diabetes Care 2002;25(7):1246–7.

[26] Centers for Disease Control and Prevention. Healthy People 2010 Focus Area 5. Diabetes Mellitus. Available at: http://www.cdc.gov/nchs/ppt/hpdata2010/focusareas/fa05_book.ppt. Accessed January 2, 2006.

[27] Winkleby MA, Kraemer HC, Ahn DK, et al. Ethnic and socioeconomic differences in cardiovascular disease risk factors: findings for women from the Third National Health and Nutrition Examination Survey, 1988,–1994. JAMA 1998;280(4):356–62.

[28] Banerji MA, Lebovitz HE. Coronary heart disease risk factor profiles in black patients with non-insulin-dependent diabetes mellitus: paradoxic patterns. Am J Med 1991;91(1):51–8.

[29] Reaven PD, Sacks J. Reduced coronary artery and abdominal aortic calcification in Hispanics with type 2 diabetes. Diabetes Care 2004;27(5):1115–20.

[30] Bild DE, Detrano R, Peterson D, et al. Ethnic differences in coronary calcification: The Multi-Ethnic Study of Atherosclerosis (MESA). Circulation 2005;111(10):1313–20.

[31] Budoff MJ, Yang TP, Shavelle RM, et al. Ethnic differences in coronary atherosclerosis. J Am Coll Cardiol 2002;39(3):408–12.

[32] Mitchell BD, Haffner SM, Hazuda HP, et al. Diabetes and coronary heart disease risk in Mexican Americans. Ann Epidemiol 1992;2(1–2):101–6.

[33] US Census Bureau Data. Available at: http://www.census.gov/ipc/www/usinterimproj/natprojtab01a.pdf. Accessed January 1, 2006.

[34] Engelgau MM, Geiss LS, Saaddine JB, et al. The evolving diabetes burden in the United States. Ann Intern Med 2004;140(11):945–50.

[35] Jones DW, Chambless LE, Folsom AR, et al. Risk factors for coronary heart disease in African Americans: The Atherosclerosis Risk in Communities Study, 1987,–1997. Arch Intern Med 2002;162(22):2565–71.

[36] Brancati FL, Kao WHL, Folsom AR, et al. Incident Type 2 Diabetes Mellitus in African American and White adults: The Atherosclerosis Risk in Communities Study. JAMA 2000;283(17):2253–9.

[37] Lee TC, O'Malley PG, Feuerstein I, et al. The prevalence and severity of coronary artery calcification on coronary artery computed tomography in black and white subjects. J Am Coll Cardiol 2003;41(1):39–44.

[38] Bonds DE, Zaccaro DJ, Karter AJ, et al. Ethnic and racial differences in diabetes care: The Insulin Resistance Atherosclerosis Study. Diabetes Care 2003;26(4):1040–6.

[39] Stern MP, Mitchell BD. Diabetes in Hispanic Americans. In: Diabetes in America. 2nd edition. Bethesda, MD: National Diabetes Data Group of the National Institute of Diabetes and Digestive and Kidney Diseases, National Institutes of Health. p. 631–660.

[40] Nelson R, Sievers M, Knowler W, et al. Low incidence of fatal coronary heart disease in Pima Indians despite high prevalence of non-insulin-dependent diabetes. Circulation 1990;81(3):987–95.

[41] Howard BV, Lee ET, Cowan LD, et al. Rising tide of cardiovascular disease in American Indians: The Strong Heart Study. Circulation 1999;99(18):2389–95.

[42] Banerji MA, Faridi N, Atluri R, et al. Body composition, visceral fat, leptin, and insulin resistance in Asian Indian men. J Clin Endocrinol Metab 1999;84(1):137–44.

[43] Raji A, Seely EW, Arky RA, et al. Body fat distribution and insulin resistance in healthy Asian Indians and Caucasians. J Clin Endocrinol Metab 2001;86(11):5366–71.

[44] Raji A, Gerhard-Herman MD, Warren M, et al. Insulin resistance and vascular dysfunction in nondiabetic Asian Indians. J Clin Endocrinol Metab 2004;89(8):3965–72.

[45] Magnus P, Beaglehole R. The real contribution of the major risk factors to the coronary epidemics: time to end the "Only-50%" myth. Arch Intern Med 2001;161(22):2657–60.

[46] Canto JG, Iskandrian AE. Major risk factors for cardiovascular disease: debunking the "Only 50%" myth. JAMA 2003;290(7):947–9.

[47] Schulze MB, Rimm EB, Li T, et al. C-Reactive protein and incident cardiovascular events among men with diabetes. Diabetes Care 2004;27(4):889–94.

[48] Mojiminiyi OA, Abdella N, Moussa MA, et al. Association of C-reactive protein with coronary heart disease risk factors in patients with type 2 diabetes mellitus. Diabetes Res Clin Pract 2002;58(1):37–44.

[49] Saito I, Folsom AR, Brancati FL, et al. Nontraditional risk factors for coronary heart disease incidence among persons with diabetes: The Atherosclerosis Risk in Communities (ARIC). Study Ann Intern Med 2000;133(2):81–91.

[50] Anand SS, Razak F, Yi Q, et al. C-Reactive protein as a screening test for cardiovascular risk in a multiethnic population. Arterioscler Thromb Vasc Biol 2004;24(8):1509–15.

[51] Forouhi NG, Sattar N, McKeigue PM. Relation of C-reactive protein to body fat distribution and features of the metabolic syndrome in Europeans and South Asians. Int J Obes Relat Metab Disord 2001;25(9):1327–31.

[52] Anand SS, Yusuf S, Vuksan V, et al. Differences in risk factors, atherosclerosis, and cardiovascular disease between ethnic groups in Canada: the Study of Health Assessment and Risk in Ethnic groups (SHARE). Lancet 2000;356(9226):279–84.

[53] Hoogeveen RC, Gambhir JK, Gambhir DS, et al. Evaluation of Lp[a] and other independent risk factors for CHD in Asian Indians and their USA counterparts. J Lipid Res 2001;42(4):631–8.

[54] Mishra A, Vikram NK. Insulin resistance syndrome (Metabolic Syndrome) and obesity in Asian Indians: evidence and implications. Nutrition 2004;20:482–91.

[55] Chandalia M, Deedwania PC. Coronary heart disease and its related risk factors in Asian Indians. Adv Exp Med Biol 2001;49:27–34.

[56] Gupta R. Burden of coronary heart disease in India. Indian Heart J 2005;57(6):632–8.

[57] Verma NP, Mehta SP, Madhu S, et al. Prevalence of known diabetes in an urban Indian environment: the Darya Ganj diabetes survey. Br Med J (Clin Res Ed) 1986;293(6544):423–4.

[58] Ramachandran A, Snehalatha C, Dharmaraj D, et al. Prevalence of glucose intolerance in Asian Indians. Urban-rural difference and significance of upper body adiposity. Diabetes Care 1992;15(10):1348–55.

[59] Bajaj M, Banerji MA. Type 2 diabetes in South Asians: a pathophysiologic focus on the Asian-Indian epidemic. Curr Diab Rep 2004;4(3):213–8.

[60] Enas EA. Coronary artery disease epidemic in Indians: a cause for alarm and call for action. J Indian Med Assoc 2000;98(11):694–5, 697–702.

[61] Uppaluri CR. Heart disease and its related risk factors in Asian Indians. Ethn Dis 2002;12(1):45–53.

[62] Abate N, Chandalia M. The impact of ethnicity on type 2 diabetes. J Diabetes Complications 2003;17:39–58.

[63] McKeigue PM, Shah B, Marmot MG. Relation of central obesity and insulin resistance with high diabetes prevalence and cardiovascular risk in South Asians. Lancet 1991;337(8738):382–6.

[64] Packard KA, Majeed F, Mohiuddin SM, et al. Low high-density lipoprotein is associated with impaired endothelial function in Asian Indians. Ethn Dis 2005;15:555–61.

[65] Becker DM, Yanek LR, Johnson WR Jr, et al. Impact of a community-based multiple risk factor intervention on cardiovascular risk in black families with a history of premature coronary disease. Circulation 2005;111(10):1298–304.

[66] Karter AJ, Ferrara A, Liu JY, et al. Ethnic disparities in diabetic complications in an insured population. JAMA 2002;287(19):2519–27.
[67] Kirk JK, Bell RA, Bertoni AG, et al. Ethnic disparities: control of glycemia, blood pressure, and LDL cholesterol among US adults with type 2 diabetes. Ann Pharmacother 2005;39(9): 1489–501.
[68] Harris MI. Racial and ethnic differences in health care access and health outcomes for adults with type 2 diabetes. Diabetes Care 2001;24(3):454–9.
[69] Adams AS, Zhang F, Mah C, et al. Race differences in long-term diabetes management in an HMO. Diabetes Care 2005;28(12):2844–9.
[70] Lanting LC, Joung IMA, Mackenbach JP, Lamberts SWJ, Bootsma AH. Ethnic Differences in Mortality, End-Stage Complications, and Quality of Care Among Diabetic Patients: A review Diabetes Care 2005;28(9):2280–88.
[71] Lanting LC, Joung IMA, Mackenbach JP, et al. Ethnic differences in mortality, end-stage complications, and quality of care among diabetic patients: a review. Diabetes Care 2005; 28(9):2280–8.
[72] Bild DE, Bluemke DA, Burke GL, et al. Multi-ethnic study of atherosclerosis: objectives and design. Am J Epidemiol 2002;156(9):871–81.
[73] Smith MW, Lautenberger JA, Shin HD, et al. Markers for mapping by admixture linkage disequilibrium in African American and Hispanic populations. Am J Hum Genet 2001; 69(5):1080–94.
[74] Flegal KM, Carroll MD, Ogden CL, et al. Prevalence and trends in obesity among US adults, 1999–2000. JAMA 2002;288(14):1723–7.
[75] Ford ES, Giles WH, Dietz WH. Prevalence of the metabolic syndrome among US adults: findings from the third National Health and Nutrition Examination Survey. JAMA 2002; 287(3):356–9.
[76] Kenny SJAR, Geiss LS. Prevalence and incidence of non-insulin-dependent diabetes. In: National Diabetes Data Group, editor. Diabetes in America. Bethesda, MD: US Dept of Health and Human Services, Public Health Service, National Institutes of Health; 1995. p. 47–68.
[77] Egede LE, Zheng D. Modifiable cardiovascular risk factors in adults with diabetes: prevalence and missed opportunities for physician counseling. Arch Intern Med 2002;162(4): 427–33.
[78] Harwell TS, Gohdes D, Moore K, et al. Cardiovascular disease and risk factors in Montana American Indians and non-Indians. Am J Prev Med 2001;20(3):196–201.
[79] McNeely MJ, Boyko EJ. Diabetes-related comorbidities in Asian Americans: results of a national health survey. J Diabetes Complications 2005;19(2):101–6.

ELSEVIER
SAUNDERS

Endocrinol Metab Clin N Am
35 (2006) 651–662

ENDOCRINOLOGY
AND METABOLISM
CLINICS
OF NORTH AMERICA

Index

Note: Page numbers of article titles are in **boldface** type.

A

ACCORD trial, 504

Action potential, prolonged, in diabetic cardiomyopathy, 580

ADHERE study, 583

Adipokines, atherosclerosis and, 526–527
  in polycystic ovarian syndrome, 617, 620

Adiponectin, atherosclerosis and, 526

Adipose tissue, peroxisome proliferator-activated receptor gamma and, 563–564

ADVANCE study, 477, 484

Advanced glycation end products (AGEs), in diabetic cardiomyopathy, 578–580, 582, 586
  in diabetic cardiovascular disease, **511–524**
    pathophysiologic evidence for, 512–513
    receptor for, 512–520. See also *Receptor for advanced glycation end products (RAGE).*
    summary overview of, 511, 520–521
  in insulin resistance, atherosclerosis with, 527–528, 535, 538, 540

African Americans, diabetic heart disease in, 635–639, 645

Aldosterone antagonists, for diabetic cardiomyopathy, 593–594
  for diabetic nephropathy, 475–476

ALLHAT study, 479, 482

ALT-711, for diabetic cardiomyopathy, 586
  for receptor for advanced glycation end products blockade, 519–520

American College of Cardiology/American Heart Association (ACC/AHA), heart failure classification of, 584

heart failure management recommendations of, 586

American Indians, diabetic heart disease in, 635–639, 645

Aminoguanidine, for receptor for advanced glycation end products blockade, 519

Amphoterin, in diabetic cardiovascular disease, receptor for advanced glycation end products and, 513–514

ANBP-2 study, 482

Androgen production, in polycystic ovarian syndrome, 612–616

Androstenedione, age-appropriate levels of, 612

AngII atherosclerosis, peroxisome proliferator-activated receptor gamma and, 565–566

Angiotensin-converting enzyme (ACE), in diabetes, hypertension and, 472–475

Angiotensin-converting enzyme 2 (ACE2), in diabetes, hypertension and, 473–475

Angiotensin-converting enzyme (ACE) inhibitors, for diabetes, as preventive, 482–483
    with heart failure, 481
    with nephropathy, 472, 475–478
  for diabetic cardiomyopathy, 588–589, 591, 606

Angiotensin II (AII), in diabetic cardiomyopathy, 583, 606
  insulin resistance and, 471

Angiotensin II type 1 receptor blockers (ARBs), for diabetes, as preventive, 482–483
    with heart failure, 481
    with nephropathy, 472, 475–478

Animal model studies, for diabetic cardiomyopathy, 578, 580, 582
  importance of, 603

0889-8529/06/$ - see front matter © 2006 Elsevier Inc. All rights reserved.
doi:10.1016/S0889-8529(06)00057-0

Moving?

Make sure your subscription moves with you!

To notify us of your new address, find your **Clinics Account Number** (located on your mailing label above your name), and contact customer service at:

E-mail: elspcs@elsevier.com

800-654-2452 (subscribers in the U.S. & Canada)
407-345-4000 (subscribers outside of the U.S. & Canada)

Fax number: 407-363-9661

Elsevier Periodicals Customer Service
6277 Sea Harbor Drive
Orlando, FL 32887-4800

*To ensure uninterrupted delivery of your subscription, please notify us at least 4 weeks in advance of move.

ELSEVIER